The Finalist's Guide to Passing the OSCE

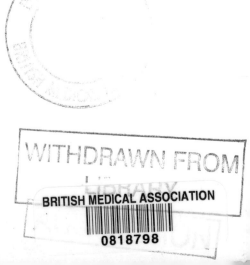

The Finalist's Guide to Passing the OSCE

CLINICAL EXAMINATIONS AND PROCEDURES

IAN MANN
MBBS, BMedSci (Hons)
Foundation Year 2 Doctor
Colchester Hospital University NHS Foundation Trust

and

ALASTAIR NOYCE
MBBS, BMedSci (Hons)
Academic Foundation Year 2 Doctor
Barts and the London NHS Trust

Foreword by
SUSAN V GELDING
Associate Dean for Undergraduates / Consultant Physician
Honorary Professor of Medical Education
Newham University Hospital London

Original line art and photographs by
MANINDER KHASRIYA
and
JOHN WONG

Radcliffe Publishing
Oxford • New York

Radcliffe Publishing Ltd
18 Marcham Road
Abingdon
Oxon OX14 1AA
United Kingdom

www.radcliffe-oxford.com
Electronic catalogue and worldwide online ordering facility.

British Library Cataloguing in Publication Data
A catalogue record for this book is available from the British Library.

ISBN-13: 978 184619 312 5

The paper used for the text pages of this book is FSC certified. FSC (The Forest Stewardship Council) is an international network to promote responsible management of the world's forests.

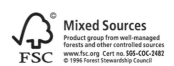

Mixed Sources
Product group from well-managed forests and other controlled sources
www.fsc.org Cert no. SGS-COC-2482
© 1996 Forest Stewardship Council

Typeset by Pindar NZ, Auckland, New Zealand
Printed and bound by TJI Digital, Padstow, Cornwall, UK

Contents

Illustrations list

Part A: Clinical examinations

Part B: Procedures

Preface

The Objective Structured Clinical Examination (OSCE) is the most daunting assessment for the medical student, particularly in the final year. Medical students are rightly expected to take full and accurate medical histories, perform structured and comprehensive clinical examinations, and display competence and dexterity when performing procedures. In doing all these tasks, they must also demonstrate interest and enthusiasm towards their patients, and show empathy when appropriate. It is natural to worry about performance and the possibility of making mistakes when under the scrutiny of observers, but good preparation and knowledge of how points are scored can do much to overcome fears.

Performing well in these exams, particularly when they involve real patients, requires a depth of medical knowledge about procedures and a systematic approach to clinical examination. Traditionally, most OSCE textbooks have attempted to cover both aspects in full, with varying degrees of success. In reality, this tends to result in either a very large textbook or, in the interests of brevity, certain topics being not fully covered. Thus, these books often fail in their primary objectives: to be simple, useful and supportive of an integrated learning approach. We believe that the ideal OSCE textbook provides details on structure and approach, whilst being of a size that lends itself to situational use: at the bedside, on the ward, or whilst observing a student colleague examining a patient. We are fortunate to live in an age where additional medical information can be obtained at the click of a mouse on a ward/personal computer, or even at the click of a button on one's mobile telephone. Why would anyone want to carry it all around in a book?

Foremost, this book provides a step-wise guide to clinical examination and to typical practical procedures, but it is written for the OSCE situation. As such, it provides details on preparation, how to approach the patient, and always concludes with information on presenting one's findings. It also, and essentially, contains example mark schemes, which indicate where points are won in the exam.

We have written this book for two main readerships: final-year medicine students who need a quick reference to clinical examination, but are already equipped with an adequate knowledge of clinical medicine, and pre-clinical and new clinical medicine students who require a blueprint to the clinical examination process.

Of course, there is no substitute for actual and repeated examination of patients, and performance of procedures, but we hope that you find this textbook the ideal adjunct to these learning experiences.

Ian Mann
Alastair Noyce
June 2009

Foreword

The undergraduate medical student must acquire a vast amount of knowledge during their training, but it is the practical exams which are the most feared. The Objective Structured Clinical Examination (OSCE) ensures that only those students who have competently acquired the techniques of clinical examination and can safely undertake practical procedures will graduate. Mastering these skills requires a firm foundation and that is exactly what this excellent book provides.

The authors should be commended on successfully combining step-by-step guidance on all the examination systems and common practical procedures in a succinct format. The manual also includes helpful tips on presenting the findings to the examiner and how the OSCE marks are awarded. Avoiding exhaustive lists of potential causes or signs so favoured by more weighty texts which tend to sit on the bookshelf unopened, this is a book that will be easy to dip into again and again whenever a student is faced with performing a particular examination or procedure.

The work benefits from being written by authors who are themselves recently familiar with the challenges of the final year OSCE. It should boost the confidence not only of junior medical students starting out in clinical examination, but also more senior students approaching their final year OSCE, junior doctors preparing for higher exams and even the senior clinicians who teach them.

Its easy to read style, packed full of handy hints, with a focus on real practice makes it an ideal companion for students and doctors alike. The guide expertly fills a void and should be greatly welcomed. This valuable book is sure to become a mainstay on the ward, in the student common room and the doctor's mess I only wish it had been available when I was a student coming up to finals!

Susan V Gelding
Associate Dean for Undergraduates / Consultant Physician
Honorary Professor of Medical Education
Newham University Hospital
London
June 2009

About the authors

Dr Ian Mann graduated from St Bartholomew's and The Royal London School of Medicine and Dentistry in 2007, with distinctions in Clinical Practice and Clinical Science. He also gained a first-class Biomedical Sciences degree with honours in Molecular Therapeutics during his intercalated year at medical school.

He is currently working at Colchester General Hospital in his second year of the Foundation Programme, and is preparing to undertake a Core Medical Training post at the Royal Brompton Hospital.

Dr Mann has a particular interest in Cardiology, as well as General and Acute Medicine. He is also interested in medical education and dedicates a large amount of his time to the ward-based teaching of medical students and nursing staff.

Dr Alastair Noyce graduated from St Bartholomew's and The Royal London School of Medicine and Dentistry in 2007, with distinctions in Medical Science, Clinical Science and Clinical Practice. He undertook an intercalated year in Molecular Therapeutics, for which he received a first-class Biomedical Sciences degree with honours, in 2006.

He is currently in the second year of an Academic Foundation Programme in North East Thames Foundation School, and is preparing to undertake an Academic Clinical Fellowship in Neurosciences at University College Hospital and the Institute of Neurology, Queen's Square. In addition to Neurology, his interests include Acute Medicine, Prescribing Errors and Patient Safety.

Dr Noyce has maintained a keen interest in teaching throughout his

Junior medical career. He has amassed considerable experience in teaching and mentoring medical students, particularly in the areas of clinical examination and academic careers in medicine.

Acknowledgements

We would like to express our sincere thanks to Maninder Khasriya and John Wong for their hard work in providing the pictures (original line art and photographs) for the book. We would also like to thank the models that posed for the photographs. They are all current medical students of St Bartholomew's and The Royal London School of Medicine and Dentistry. We are grateful to the clinicians who kindly reviewed the subject matter and their names are listed below by way of recognition. Finally, we would like to extend our thanks to St Bartholomew's and The Royal London School of Medicine and Dentistry for allowing us to use their excellent Clinical Skills Centre, whilst compiling this book.

Content review

Dr Sandip Banerjee, Specialist Registrar in Respiratory Medicine
Dr Rachel Farrell, Specialist Registrar in Neurology
Professor Susan Gelding, Consultant in Endocrinology and Diabetes
Dr Noor Jawad, Specialist Registrar in Gastroenterology
Dr Nikesh Malik, Specialist Registrar in Cardiology
Mr Faisal Mihaimeed, Consultant in Breast, Thyroid and General Surgery
Dr Andrew Rochford, Specialist Registrar in Gastroenterology
Dr Arjune Sen, Specialist Registrar in Neurology
Dr Ferdinand Von Walden, Muscle Physiologist and Medical Doctor

Modelo

Aaron Braddy

Richard Donovan

Sonya Gadhvi

Shahrzad Hadavi

Sabra Pechrak Manesh

Vanessa Watkins

Jeeves Wijesuriya

Abbreviations

ABG	arterial blood gas
ABPI	ankle–brachial pressure index
AF	atrial fibrillation
BMI	body mass index
BP	blood pressure
CN	cranial nerve
CT	computed tomography (scan)
DIP	distal interphalangeal (joint)
DRE	digital rectal examination
DVT	deep vein thrombosis
ECG	electrocardiogram
FNAC	fine needle aspiration for cytology
GALS	gait, arms, legs, spine
GI	gastrointestinal
IV	intravenous
JPS	joint position sensation
JVP	jugular venous pulsation
LMN	lower motor neurone
MCP	metacarpophalangeal (joint)
NGT	nasogastric tube
OSCE	objective structured clinical examination
PEG	percutaneous endoscopic gastrostomy
PEFR	peak expiratory flow rate
PIP	proximal interphalangeal (joint)
RAPD	relative afferent pupillary defect

SFJ	saphenofemoral junction
UMN	upper motor neurone

Part A

Clinical examinations

Cardiovascular

Introduction

When conducting an examination of the cardiovascular system, it is impera-
tive that one thinks systematically. As you elicit signs, these should be used
to formulate your differential diagnosis. For example, if you discover early
that the patient has an irregular pulse, look further for reasons as to why.
Do they have the murmur of mitral stenosis, causing them to be in atrial
fibrillation (AF) secondary to a dilated left atrium? Thinking systematically
allows you to organise your differential and structure your case presentation
to the examiner upon completion.

Before you start

Enter the station and read the instructions carefully. When you are satisfied
with the station requirements, introduce yourself to the patient and the
examiner, if you have not yet done so. Explain the examination to the patient
and gain their verbal consent. Wash your hands and position yourself at the
end of the bed.

Patient position is crucial to the cardiovascular examination. The ideal
position is with the patient semi-recumbent at 45°. You can position the
patient at the beginning of the examination or during it, but indicate this to
the examiner. Ensure that the patient is comfortable and adequately exposed,
as well as adequately covered.

This whole process should take about 30 seconds, but try not to dwell on
it for greater than 1 minute.

Examination

General

This should be conducted initially from the end of the bed. Ask yourself:
- Does the patient look well or unwell?
- Are they comfortable at rest or are they in pain/distress?
- Are they short of breath?
- Do they have any scars (chest and legs)?
- Are there paraphernalia around the bed that indicate their underlying illness, e.g. medications (including sublingual nitrates), oxygen and cardiac-monitoring equipment?

The hands and arms

From the right-hand side of the patient, ask them to extend their hands. Look for:
- clubbing (causes include bacterial endocarditis, congenital cyanotic heart disease)
- tar staining
- capillary refill – press the nail bed for five seconds and release. Refill should occur in less than two seconds
- peripheral cyanosis
- peripheral stigmata of infective endocarditis (splinter haemorrhages, Janeway lesions and Osler's nodes)
- palmar erythema (high-output states)
- pallor of the palmar creases (indicative of anaemia)
- tendon xanthomata.

Do not attempt to mention all of the above. Three or four peripheral signs should suffice. It is more important to make your examination of the hands purposeful and structured, so that you acknowledge signs, if indeed they are present.

Make an assessment of the radial pulse. Pass comment on the following, if you feel able:
- rate (normal pulse rate is 60–100 beats per minute)
- regularity
- symmetry
- collapsing pulse (aortic regurgitation) – check that they have no pain in their shoulder and warn of what you are going to do

- volume and character (it may only be possible to determine these from a central pulse).

One should compare sides for radial–radial delay, and also at the groin for radial–femoral delay.

Blood pressure – in most cases it is sufficient to ask the examiner for this. Be mindful of:
- pulse pressure – wide versus narrow
- postural hypotension
- symmetry (check whether the right arm blood pressure is the same as that of the left).

The face and neck
Eyes should be checked for:
- corneal arcus
- xanthelasma
- pallor of the conjunctiva.

Comment on the presence or absence of mitral facies.

Ask the patient to open their mouth. Look for:
- poor dentition
- central cyanosis.

The carotid pulses should be palpated one side at a time. It may be easier to pass comment on pulse character and volume from this central position.
   Examination of the jugular venous pulsation (JVP) should begin by ensuring that the patient is reclined at 45°. Further position the patient by gently turning their head away from you and ensuring that it is supported by the pillow or couch. One should ensure that the sternocleidomastoid muscles are as relaxed as possible. The course of the internal jugular vein becomes visible between the two heads of the muscle and runs posterior to the lobe of the ear. Look along this line for evidence of a visible, double pulsation. Once identified, attempt to palpate. If it is the JVP, it will not be palpable. Ask the patient if they have any abdominal pain and warn them that you are going to press down on their abdomen. If agreed, press gently

but firmly over the liver and watch for transient rising of the pulsation. It will subsequently fall if pressure is removed or sustained (providing adequately hydrated). Finally, assess the height of the JVP (the vertical height from the angle of Louis).

The praecordium
Start with the anterior chest wall and work through the following before asking the patient to sit forward to allow you to examine their back.

Inspection
Comment on:
- presence/absence of scars (e.g. sternotomy or thoracotomy scars)
- chest wall deformity
- visible pulsation.

Palpation
Feel for:
- the apex beat (left mid-clavicular line, 5th intercostal space) and comment if deviated from this. One can also comment on its character (e.g. tapping, sustained)
- heaves (from the right ventricle) or thrills (palpable murmurs)
- a pacemaker (which may be visible in patients with a low body mass index (BMI)).

Percussion
There is little to percuss in the cardiovascular examination. However, one may wish to percuss the lung bases to identify a pleural effusion, and one may also wish to percuss the liver borders if clinical evidence is found of right heart failure.

Auscultation (see Figure A1.1)
You must develop a system for this, as it is the most complicated part of the cardiovascular examination. It is easy to confuse yourself and give the impression that you have had no experience with auscultation. Listen with the diaphragm of your stethoscope unless otherwise indicated.

You should listen at the:

- apex/mitral area – place your stethoscope wherever you feel the apex beat (use the diaphragm and the bell)
- tricuspid area – left sternal border, 4th intercostal space
- pulmonary area – left sternal border, 2nd intercostal space
- aorta area – right sternal border, 2nd intercostal space
- carotids (listen for bruits or radiation of a murmur from the aortic valve).

Listen for:
- murmurs – systolic versus diastolic. Time a murmur with your thumb on the carotid pulsation in order to decipher whether it is systolic or diastolic. The carotid pulsation occurs at the same time as the S1 heart sound (onset of systole). Listen for evidence of radiation at the carotids and axilla.

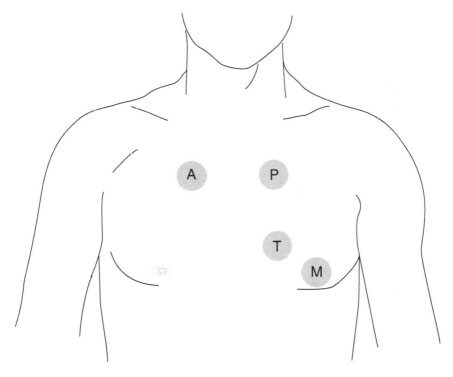

FIGURE A1.1 Areas for auscultation of the heart valves. Aortic valve (A), mitral valve (M), pulmonary valve (P), tricuspid valve (T)

- heart sounds – certain conditions alter the volume of the first and second heart sounds. Listen for splitting of the second heart sound, physiological or otherwise. Listen for third or fourth heart sounds and know the meaning of these.

The following manoeuvres will help in identification of murmurs:
- full inspiration – will emphasise physiological splitting of the second heart sound and exaggerate right-sided heart murmurs (tricuspid and pulmonary)
- full expiration – will align the aortic and pulmonary components of the second heart sound and exaggerate left-side heart murmurs (mitral and aortic)
- left lateral position – hold the stethoscope over the apex of the heart and ask the patient to roll onto their left side. This brings the mitral valve closer to your stethoscope and emphasises mitral murmurs and radiation to the axilla. Use the bell of the stethoscope to auscultate for a murmur of mitral stenosis, and the diaphragm for mitral regurgitation
- leaning forwards, auscultating at the lower left sternal edge – emphasises a regurgitant murmur across the aortic valve. Use the diaphragm to auscultate, whilst the patient is in full expiration.

The back
Once you have completed your examination of the praecordium, ask the patient to lean forward so that you can assess the posterior chest wall (the patient may already be sitting forward from your auscultation of the anterior chest wall). It is particularly important to auscultate the lung bases and listen for the characteristic crackles of pulmonary oedema. You may also percuss the lung bases for evidence of effusion (*see* above). Feel for sacral oedema, and invite the patient to recline back again. Check that they are comfortable and adequately covered.

The legs and other peripheral pulses
You should include:
- a general comment on the colour and temperature of the feet, presence of ulcers, and capillary refill
- assessment of the pulses in the feet (posterior tibial and dorsalis pedis)

- comment on the presence or absence of peripheral oedema, and how far it extends
- a final check that there are no scars that may have been missed earlier in the examination.

Completing your examination

Depending on your findings, you may wish to assess the size and pulsatility of the liver, and examine the abdominal aorta, and the femoral arterial pulsation. Thank the patient and cover them appropriately (if not already done). Wash your hands.

Comment that, in order to complete your examination, you would request a 12-lead electrocardiogram (ECG), a blood pressure (BP) check in both arms and a temperature chart. You might also mention a urine dipstick and fundoscopy.

Conclusion and presentation

Spend a couple of moments gathering your thoughts and considering your delivery to the examiner. Present the pertinent positive and negative findings that have led you to your diagnosis (or differential).

An example of your presentation may be:

> This well-looking, 70-year-old gentleman is sitting comfortably at rest. There are no paraphernalia around the bed indicating why this gentleman may be in hospital. There are no peripheral stigmata of cardiovascular disease. His pulse rate is 68 beats per minute and regular. The pulse is of low volume and appears to be slow rising. The blood pressure of 118/95 indicates a narrow pulse pressure. On inspection of the chest, I can see a well-healed sternotomy scar. There is also a scar on the medial aspect of the right leg, indicating venous harvesting. The apex beat is in the 5th intercostal space, mid-clavicular line. There is a loud ejection systolic murmur best heard in the aortic area in expiration that radiates to the carotids. The lung bases are clear, and there is no peripheral oedema. These findings are consistent with a gentleman who has undergone a coronary artery bypass graft and who also has a murmur of aortic stenosis. There are no signs of heart failure or endocarditis.

Example of a cardiovascular examination mark scheme

Before you start
- Makes introduction (full name and role)
- Offers explanation and seeks consent
- Ensures adequate exposure and patient comfort
- Ensures patient is at 45°, adequately exposed and comfortable
- Washes hands

Examination
General
- Comments on general appearance

The hands and arms
- Examines for peripheral stigmata of cardiovascular disease
- Examines radial pulse and passes comment on rate and rhythm
- Checks for radial–radial delay and radial–femoral delay
- Checks for a collapsing pulse, first ensuring that there is no pain in the shoulder
- States intention to take the blood pressure

The face and neck
- Examines the eyes and mouth for evidence of cardiovascular disease
- Examines the jugular venous pulsation with the patient at 45° and the head supported
- Examines the carotid pulse bilaterally, commenting on volume, character and symmetry

The praecordium
- Inspects the praecordium
- Palpates for the apex beat, determining its position and character
- Palpates for heaves and thrills
- Auscultates for murmurs in the mitral, tricuspid, pulmonary and aortic areas

- Times cardiac cycle with carotid pulse during auscultation
- Performs cardiovascular examination manoeuvres correctly
- Auscultates both carotids for radiation of murmurs and bruits
- Auscultates the lung bases, commenting on any signs of heart failure
- Feels for sacral oedema

The legs
- Makes general comment on the colour, temperature of feet, scars from venous harvesting
- Palpates peripheral pulses
- Assesses for peripheral oedema, stating the level

Completing your examination
- Covers the patient, ensuring that they are comfortable
- States the need for further bedside tests
- Thanks patient
- Washes hands
- Demonstrates empathy
- Presents examination findings in a concise and confident manner
- Offers (differential) diagnosis
- Does the above in a fluent, professional manner

2

Respiratory

Introduction

Respiratory disease is common and, as such, the patient load is heavy. Whereas you may not regularly carry out all the examinations discussed in this book, you will conduct a respiratory examination on the vast majority of your patients.

It is relatively easy to become complacent when performing this examination. It is not uncommon that individuals will restrict themselves to an examination either of the anterior or of the posterior chest. This is mostly unacceptable, and a thorough examination of the respiratory system will necessitate examination of both the anterior and the posterior aspects of the chest.

There are many peripheral stigmata of respiratory disease that you should be familiar with. It is important that you know the causes of these clinical signs, as they will help you to formulate your diagnosis.

Before you start

Read the instructions and make sure that you are comfortable with what is being asked of you. Enter the station and introduce yourself to both the patient and the examiner. Explain to the patient what the examination entails and gain verbal consent. Wash your hands. Patient comfort is important; they should be slightly reclined or perched on the edge of the couch. Ensure that you have the patient's chest exposed adequately.

Examination

General

Stand at the foot of the bed. Ask yourself:

- Does the patient look well or unwell?
- Are they comfortable at rest or in respiratory distress/using accessory muscles to breathe? Comment on the presence or absence of pursed-lip breathing.
- Can they speak? Can they complete sentences?
- Do they look cyanosed?
- Are they on oxygen?
- Are there visible scars or chest drains?
- Are there paraphernalia around the bed indicating the underlying illness, e.g. inhalers, nebulisers, peak flow meters, oxygen masks, sputum pots? If you see a sputum pot, be sure to examine its contents as this may give you clues to an underlying pathology.

Count the patient's respiratory rate. A normal adult respiratory rate is 12–18 breaths per minute.

The hands and arms

Move to a new position at the patient's right side. Look at their hands for:

- clubbing (causes include lung cancer, tuberculosis, bronchiectasis)
- tar staining
- wasting of the intrinsic muscles of the hands (apical lung cancers)
- peripheral cyanosis
- pallor of the palmar creases (indicative of anaemia, which may cause breathlessness).

Ask the patient to stretch their arms out, palms down. Observe for a fine tremor associated with salbutamol use. With their arms still out, ask them to cock their wrists, so that their fingers point upwards. Observe for a carbon dioxide retention flap. Mention to the examiner that, under ideal circumstances, you would observe for 30 seconds.

Palpate the radial pulse. Comment on the rate, and the presence or absence of a bounding character, which can be associated with the retention of carbon dioxide.

The face and neck

Inspect the face carefully for:

- Horner's syndrome (associated with ipsilateral apical lung cancers)
  — ptosis
  — anhydrosis
  — miosis
  — enophthalmos
- pursed-lip breathing – comment if you have not already done so (*see* above)
- pallor of the conjunctiva – gently pull down on the patient's lower eyelid.

Ask the patient to open their mouth and lift their tongue. Pass comment on the presence or absence of central cyanosis.

Check the position of the trachea using a single finger. Place the index and ring fingers on the medial part of the clavicle on either side, and use the middle finger to assess the position of the trachea. Warn the patient prior to doing so, as this may be uncomfortable. A normal trachea should pass in the midline down the anterior aspect of the neck, though in some cases it may be angled slightly to the right.

In examining the neck, it is important to assess for lymphadenopathy. This can be undertaken at any point in the examination, but it is important not to overlook it. Remember to palpate for the following lymph node collections: anterior and posterior cervical chain, pre- and post-auricular, occipital, sub-mandibular, and supra-clavicular. Examination for lymphadenopathy in the neck should be undertaken whilst standing behind the patient. Remember to warn them before touching their neck.

The chest

Start with the anterior chest wall before asking your patient to sit forward, so you can examine the posterior chest wall.

Inspection

Comment on:

- presence/absence of scars (e.g. thoracotomy, chest drain scars)
- chest wall deformities (e.g. pectus excavatum, pectus carinatum, barrel chest)

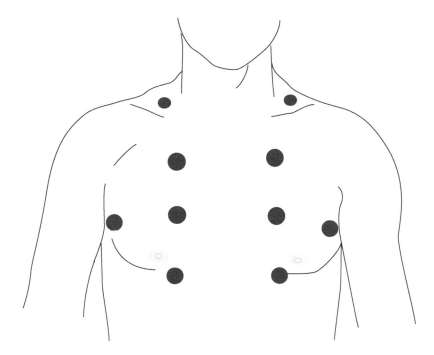

FIGURE A2.1 Areas for percussion and auscultation of the lungs

- symmetry of chest wall movement – ask the patient to take a deep breath. The side that moves less is the diseased side
- intercostal recession and paradoxical movement of the abdomen
- dilated neck veins (due to superior vena cava obstruction with apical lung tumours).

Palpation

Having observed chest expansion, you must now feel for expansion. Place your hands on either side of the anterior chest wall, with your finger curling around the chest laterally, and your thumbs approximated in the midline. Your thumbs should be held just over the sternum, without touching it. Squeeze the chest gently, so that your thumbs almost meet in the middle. Ask the patient to take a deep breath in, and observe how your thumbs separate.

Pass comment on:

- symmetry/asymmetry
- approximate number of centimetres of chest expansion.

15

Repeat the technique for the upper and lower parts of the chest.

Feel for the apex beat. Normally, this is in the left mid-clavicular line, 5th intercostal space. Displacement may occur with mediastinal shift, in which case the trachea may also be deviated.

Percussion

When percussing the chest wall, you should not only be listening to the sound, but also 'feeling' it.

Start with percussion over the clavicles. You can tap directly onto the clavicle, however, this should be done gently as it can be uncomfortable. Work your way down the chest wall percussing systematically and comparing sides. Percuss in three or four places, down both sides of the anterior chest wall. Also percuss the lateral chest walls and up towards the axillae, still comparing sides.

Pass comment on the percussion note, which may be:

- resonant
- hyper-resonant (pneumothorax)
- dull (consolidation)
- stony dull (pleural effusion).

Auscultation (see Figure A2.1)

Use the diaphragm of the stethoscope unless otherwise specified. Ask your patient to take deep breaths in and out through an open mouth.

Listen to the following areas:

- supra-clavicular fossa (the lung apex) – use the bell of the stethoscope
- level of approximately the 2nd rib
- level of approximately the 5th rib
- level of approximately the 7th rib
- mid-axillary line – be sure to ask your patient to move their arm up, so that the examiner can see what you are auscultating.

Pass comment on:

- depth of inspiration
- length of inspiratory phase compared to expiratory phase
- breath sounds (equal on both sides or reduced on one side of the chest)
- quality of breath sounds (vesicular or bronchial breathing)

- added sounds (e.g. wheeze, crackles)
- if crackles were present:
  — whether they were coarse or fine
  — whether they were timed with inspiration or expiration
  — the site of crackles.

If crackles are heard, it is important to ask the patient to cough, as the crackles might disappear afterwards. This will help to separate pathological from non-pathological crackles.

Vocal resonance and tactile vocal fremitus

Vocal resonance and tactile vocal fremitus are two methods of assessing the same thing, namely the way in which sound is transmitted through the lung parenchyma. Fremitus is a palpable vibration that is felt whilst the patient speaks. The vibration is felt by placing the ulnar border of both hands simultaneously on either side of the patient's chest wall.

Vocal resonance is the sound produced if one auscultates whilst the patient speaks. It is important to be familiar with both techniques, although it is only necessary to demonstrate one in most exam situations.

For both techniques, ask the patient to say 'ninety-nine' while listening to/palpating the same areas that were used when previously auscultating the chest. Listen/feel for the vibration, which may be:

- normal
- increased (consolidation)
- decreased (effusions and pneumothorax).

Posterior chest wall

Your examination of the posterior chest wall should mirror that of the anterior chest wall, and therefore cover the following:

- inspection
- palpation – repeat chest expansion
- percussion – do this medial to the scapulae, as they will interfere with the percussion note
- auscultation – although all parts of the chest should be given equal attention, it is important to remember that frequently signs are picked up at the lung bases.

Palpate for lymphadenopathy, if you have not already done so, and perform tactile vocal fremitus/vocal resonance.

Whilst examining the posterior chest, the following important points should be noted.

- Inspect the spine for scoliosis or kyphosis. Scoliosis is particularly important, as it may affect respiration, or be the result of pneumonectomy/lobectomy many years ago.
- When percussing and auscultating, you can ask your patient to cross their arms in front of them. This will move the scapulae out of the way, exposing more of the chest wall, to aid your examination.

The legs

After you have finished examining the chest, be sure to cover the patient adequately before inspecting the legs.

Assess the legs for peripheral oedema. If present, you should indicate to the examiner that you would also do a cardiovascular examination.

Completing your examination

Thank the patient. Ensure that they are left comfortable and appropriately covered. Wash your hands. Comment that, in order to complete your examination, you would request a temperature, spirometry/peak expiratory flow rate (PEFR), pulse oximetry and inspect the contents of any sputum pot.

Conclusion and presentation

Take a few moments to gather your thoughts before presenting your findings to the examiner. You must remember to present any pertinent positive and negative findings that have aided you in formulating a diagnosis, together with an appropriate differential.

An example of your presentation may be:

> This is a slim, 68-year-old lady who is sitting up in bed and is currently on 2 litres of oxygen per minute via nasal specs. Although she appears to be relatively comfortable at rest, I note that she is demonstrating pursed-lip breathing. There is no use of accessory muscles. Her respiratory rate is at the upper normal limit, currently at 20 breaths per minute. There is a nebuliser at the bedside and an inhaler containing tiotropium. Tar staining is present

on the right hand. She has a carbon dioxide retention flap and a bounding pulse. There is no evidence of cyanosis. Chest expansion is poor, at barely 1 cm, although it appears to be equal. The percussion note of the chest is resonant throughout. There is marked poor air entry throughout, with a widespread mild polyphonic wheeze and a prolonged expiratory phase of the respiratory cycle. These clinical findings are consistent with a diagnosis of chronic obstructive pulmonary disease. To complete my examination, I would like to know the oxygen saturations, perform spirometry and inspect any sputum expectorated.

Example of a respiratory examination mark scheme

Before you start
- Makes introduction (full name and role)
- Offers explanation and seeks consent
- Ensures adequate exposure and patient's comfort
- Washes hands

Examination
General
- Comments on general appearance
- Counts respiratory rate

The hands and arms
- Examines for peripheral stigmata of respiratory disease
- Examines for a carbon dioxide retention flap
- Palpates the radial pulse for a bounding pulse

The face and neck
- Examines the face for evidence of respiratory disease
- Assesses for central cyanosis
- Checks position of trachea
- Examines for lymphadenopathy

The chest

- Inspects the chest wall for scars, deformities and symmetry of movement
- Assesses chest expansion
- Correctly percusses chest wall
- Auscultates chest wall in correct manner and passes comment on findings
- Assesses either vocal resonance or tactile vocal fremitus
- Examines anterior and posterior chest

The legs

- Assesses for peripheral oedema, stating the level

Completing your examination

- Covers the patient, ensuring that they are comfortable
- States need for further bedside tests
- Thanks patient
- Washes hands
- Demonstrates empathy
- Presents examination findings in a concise and confident manner
- Offers (differential) diagnosis
- Does the above in a fluent, professional manner

3

Abdominal

Introduction

The abdominal examination (like the respiratory exam) conforms well to the typical clinical examination structure. One starts with inspection, follows with palpation and completes with percussion and auscultation. In theory, it is very simple to conduct. It is, however, difficult to make it look polished. It is easy for an examiner to spot those who have experience in examining the abdomen and those who have learnt it from a book but never practised on a patient. You also give yourself away if you ask the patient to sit up and lie flat multiple times during the course of the examination. It really doesn't matter what position the patient starts in; just remember that they ought to be sitting forward when examining the neck for lymphadenopathy, and they must be fully reclined and completely at ease when you lay your hands on their abdomen.

Before you start

Enter the station and read your instructions carefully. In some stations you may be asked to perform an abdominal examination without examining the head or chest, so be careful not to waste valuable time. Introduce yourself to the patient and the examiner. Explain to the patient what you wish to do, and gain their verbal consent. Wash your hands and assume a position at the end of the bed. Patient comfort and relaxation are absolutely essential for the abdominal exam, and this may shape how you position and expose the patient from the outset. Ideally, the patient will be lying flat and be exposed from 'nipples to knees', although in the context of an OSCE this might not be possible. You should at least state this to the examiner.

Examination

General

From the end of the bed you ought to comment on the following:
- Does the patient look well or unwell?
- Is the patient comfortable or are they in pain/distress?
- Are they jaundiced?
- Do they have any tattoos?
- Is there evidence of abdominal distention or cachexia?
- Are there obvious stigmata of chronic liver disease (*see* below)?
- Are there paraphernalia alluding to their condition, e.g. energy supplement drinks, a percutaneous endoscopic gastrostomy (PEG) feeding tube, a nasogastric tube (NGT)?

The hands and arms

Adopt a new position at the right side of the patient. Ask them to extend their hands. Look for:
- clubbing (causes include chronic liver disease, inflammatory bowel disease)
- palmar erythema
- Dupuytren's contracture
- leuconychia
- koilonychia
- asterixis – the patient should have their arms extended and their hands cocked at the wrist. Ideally they should hold this position for 30 seconds
- ecchymoses
- excoriations
- track marks (intravenous drug users)
- arteriovenous fistulae.

The face and mouth

The eyes should be examined by gently pulling down on the lower lid and looking for:

- icteric sclera (jaundice)
- pallor of the conjunctiva (may herald the finding of anaemia in the patient).

Ask the patient to open their mouth. Clinical findings may include:
- poor dentition
- ulceration (aphthous or otherwise) – ask the patient to pull down their lower lip
- glossitis
- angular stomatitis
- labial changes in pigmentation
- the smell of ketones, or fetor hepaticus.

Finally, comment on the presence/absence of parotid gland enlargement.

The neck, chest and back

To reiterate, this is often where one demonstrates just how often one has been through this examination process. We recommend having the patient sit up during this phase of the examination. However, they may start the examination reclined, for comfort's sake.

Start with the chest. Look for:
- gynaecomastia (and feel for glandular tissue)
- abnormal hair distribution
- spider naevi (more than five in the distribution of the superior vena cava).

Ask the patient to sit forward, whilst you move to a position behind them. Check the back for spider naevi and for a buffalo hump or acanthosis nigricans. Palpate along the length of the cervical chain, pre- and post-auricular, occipital, submandibular and supraclavicular lymph nodes. Pay particular attention to the left supraclavicular fossa, and pass comment on the Virchow's node.

The abdomen

Inspection

Ask the patient to lie on their back, hands by their sides, and then adjust the couch to ensure that they are lying flat. Inspect the abdomen more closely.

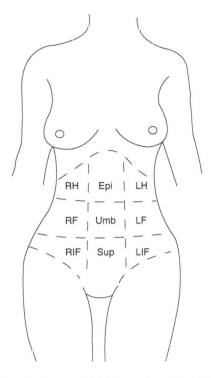

FIGURE A3.1 Areas of the abdomen. Right hypochondrium (RH), epigastrium (Epi), left hypochondrium (LH), right flank (RF), umbilical (Umb), left flank (LF), right iliac fossa (RIF), suprapubic (Sup), left iliac fossa (LIF)

Comment on:
- movement – is it rising and falling with respiration?
- scars – remember to look at the flanks and hernial orifices
- distention (symmetrical versus asymmetrical)
- visible peristalsis
- caput medusae
- visible masses, including hernias.

Palpation

Ask the patient if they have any pain. If yes, ask them to point to the area with a single finger. Ask them to cough. Does this make the pain any worse? Look carefully when the patient coughs, since the transient rise in intra-abdominal pressure may cause a hernia to expose itself. Warm your hands whilst you observe.

Ensure that, before you begin palpation, you crouch or kneel so that you are at eye-level with the patient's abdomen. Start palpation away from the painful area. When palpating, you must always look at the patient's face, and try to establish if there is:

- tenderness
- guarding
- rebound tenderness
- an abdominal mass.

Starting gently, palpate all nine areas of the abdomen in a systematic manner, taking care not to miss any (*see* Figure A3.1). If there is no area of tenderness, repeat your palpation in a deeper fashion, again taking care to examine all nine areas (warn the patient that you are going to push more firmly). The patient may report tenderness or, if severe, may demonstrate guarding. This is involuntary contraction of the abdominal muscles. Rebound tenderness is a sign of peritoneal inflammation and occurs when removing the hand from the abdomen suddenly. If any masses are discovered on palpation, one should describe these as one would any mass (*see* Chapter A6, Lumps and bumps).

The liver can be enlarged, or appear enlarged in a number of disease states. Palpate the liver using the blade of an inverted hand (the border of the index finger). Start in the right iliac fossa and move up to the lower border of the ribs. Time your palpation so that you are pressing in and superiorly as the patient takes a deep breath in. This will push the liver down as you move your hand up, and theoretically, if enlarged, the lower border of the liver and your hand will meet.

One should attempt to comment further on an enlarged liver, stating:

- whether it has a regular or irregular border
- whether it is pulsatile or non-pulsatile
- whether it is tender or not
- by how many fingerbreadths it is enlarged (one can use percussion of the chest to identify the superior border of the liver).

The spleen is palpated in much the same way, using the same hand technique, and starting in the right iliac fossa. This time, however, work towards the left lower rib border. Again, use the patient's deep breathing to increase the likelihood of feeling the spleen. You can ask the patient to roll towards

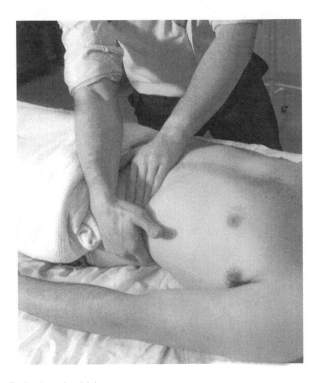

FIGURE A3.2 Balloting the kidney

you in order to improve your chances of palpating an enlarged spleen.

Kidneys are palpated using a different technique, known as balloting (*see* Figure A3.2). Slide one hand beneath the patient and into the renal angle, gently pushing up. Place the other hand on the abdomen directly above the first hand and push in towards it. Picture the kidney between your hands, and gently and repetitively push the fingers of the lower hand towards your upper hand, in an attempt to bounce the kidney against the upper hand. This should be done in inspiration. Repeat this action on the other side.

It may be necessary to demonstrate palpation of the abdominal aorta (in the epigastric area) and the bladder (in the suprapubic area).

Percussion

The use of percussion is three-fold in the abdominal exam:

- to elicit the exact size of either the liver or spleen once it has been palpated, and if it is thought to be enlarged

- to elicit tenderness consistent with peritoneal irritation
- to elicit the presence of intra-abdominal fluid/ascites (demonstration of shifting dullness).

To elicit shifting dullness, start percussion in the midline of the abdomen (where the percussion note should be resonant) and percuss down towards the right flank. When the percussion note becomes dull, percuss accurately to determine where the interface between resonant and dull is. Mark this point with your middle finger. Invite the patient to turn away from you, onto their side, keeping your finger where the difference in percussion note was heard.

Keep them on their side for longer than 30 seconds, and then percuss again. The percussion note of the point at which you marked may have become resonant. With the patient still on their side, percuss down towards the midline of the abdomen until the percussion note becomes dull again, i.e. a shift in the 'dullness'. Demonstration of this sign is consistent with a finding of intra-abdominal fluid.

Auscultation

Auscultation should be performed near the end of the exam. Pick a spot on the abdomen, often to one side of the umbilicus, and place the diaphragm of the stethoscope gently on the skin. Bowel sounds should be heard in the normal abdomen. They may be normal, tinkling, scanty, hyperactive or absent.

Also take the opportunity to auscultate for renal bruits. To do this, place the stethoscope above and lateral to the umbilicus (remember that the abdominal aorta bifurcates to become the common iliac arteries at the umbilicus).

Completing your examination

No abdominal examination is complete without offering to examine the external genitalia, the hernial orifices, and performing a digital rectal examination (DRE) and urinalysis. However, in most OSCE scenarios it is sufficient to simply mention these.

One should also remember to check for pedal oedema, which can occur in low-protein states.

Cover the patient appropriately, thank them and return them to a position of comfort on the couch. Wash your hands.

Conclusion and presentation

Collect your thoughts in preparation for presentation, and formulate a differential diagnosis. A confident examination presentation may be:

> This is a middle-aged Asian gentleman, who appears comfortable at rest. Peripherally there is evidence of chronic liver disease, which includes clubbing and leuconychia. He has asterixis and is icteric. There are four spider naevi on the anterior chest wall and three on the posterior chest wall. His abdomen is distended but non-tender. I cannot palpate the liver, but the spleen appears to extend 3 cm past the left costal margin. The percussion note is dull towards the flanks, and there is shifting dullness. These findings, including jaundice, encephalopathy and ascites, are consistent with a diagnosis of decompensated chronic liver disease with evidence of portal hypertension. To complete my abdominal examination, I would like to perform a digital rectal examination, examine the hernial orifices and perform urinalysis.

Example of an abdominal examination mark scheme

Before you start
- Makes introduction (full name and role)
- Offers explanation and seeks consent
- Ensures adequate exposure and patient's comfort
- Positions patient appropriately for each examination stage
- Washes hands

Examination

General
- Comments on general appearance

The hands and arms
- Examines for peripheral stigmata of gastrointestinal/liver disease
- Examines for asterixis

The face and mouth
- Examines the eyes for jaundice
- Undertakes appropriate examination of the mouth

The neck, chest and back
- Looks for stigmata of gastrointestinal/liver disease
- Palpates for lymphadenopathy

The abdomen
- Makes focused inspection of the abdomen
- Enquires about pain
- Palpates lightly in nine areas of the abdomen
- Palpates deeply in nine areas of the abdomen (if appropriate)
- Palpates for the liver using the correct technique
- Palpates for the spleen using the correct technique
- Ballots for the kidneys
- Uses percussion appropriately to further characterise organomegaly
- Demonstrates 'shifting dullness' technique
- Auscultates for bowel sounds

Completing your examination
- Covers the patient, ensuring that they are comfortable
- States need for further examinations and bedside tests
- Thanks patient
- Washes hands
- Demonstrates empathy
- Presents examination findings in a concise and confident manner
- Offers (differential) diagnosis
- Does the above in a fluent, professional manner

4

Cranial nerves

Introduction

Examining the cranial nerves is a simple but strangely daunting task for students. An accomplished examination necessitates a basic understanding of the neurological anatomy and a good deal of practice. You will make your life much easier if you can interchange between referring to the given number of the cranial nerve (CN) and its actual name (or branch).

CRANIAL NERVE NUMBER	ACTUAL NAME	MAIN FUNCTIONS
Cranial nerve I	Olfactory nerve	Smell – sensory
Cranial nerve II	Optic nerve	Sight – sensory
Cranial nerve III	Oculomotor nerve	Eye movements – motor
Cranial nerve IV	Trochlear nerve	Adducts the depressed eye – motor
Cranial nerve V	Trigeminal nerve	Mastication and facial sensation – motor and sensory
Cranial nerve VI	Abducens nerve	Abducts the eye – motor
Cranial nerve VII	Facial nerve	Facial movements and taste (anterior two-thirds of the tongue) – motor and sensory
Cranial nerve VIII	Vestibulocochlear nerve	Hearing and balance – sensory
Cranial nerve IX	Glossopharyngeal nerve	Swallowing and taste (posterior third of the tongue) – motor and sensory
Cranial nerve X	Vagus nerve	Swallowing and autonomic function – motor, sensory and autonomic
Cranial nerve XI	Accessory nerve	Neck movements – motor
Cranial nerve XII	Hypoglossal nerve	Tongue movements – motor

Above is a list of the cranial nerves and their main functions. It is not exhaustive and represents the bare minimum knowledge that one should be equipped with for a cranial nerves examination. Many of the nerves have a number of other functions that the high-scoring student should be aware of. For those who are looking for a more complete understanding, it is worth learning the origins, course and destination of each nerve, and the foramina from which they emerge in the skull.

You have two choices when examining the cranial nerves. Most candidates will examine in numerical order, starting with CN I and testing through to CN XII. A handful of candidates will test cranial nerves according to the anatomy and modify their examination as they build a picture of the diagnosis. This allows one to generate hypotheses whilst examining and then to test these hypotheses. However, since the majority of candidates will examine based on the premise that CN I comes first, followed by CN II, followed by CN III etc, we will cater accordingly.

Before you start

Enter the station and read your instructions carefully. Introduce yourself to the patient and explain what you want to do, e.g. 'I have been asked to test the nerves in your head.' Gain their verbal consent and position them appropriately.

When examining the cranial nerves, the patient can be lying semi-recumbent on the couch or sat on the edge. Remember to wash your hands thoroughly.

Examination

General

Standing at a short distance, observe for the following:
- a facial/VIIth nerve palsy (signified by facial drooping)
- abnormalities in conjugate gaze/strabismus
- spontaneous facial movements, e.g. swallowing, blinking
- abnormal movements, e.g. tics
- abnormalities involving the rest of body, e.g. abnormal posturing, appearance consistent with a hemiparesis.

The cranial nerves

Cranial nerve I – olfactory nerve

This is difficult to test in the context of an OSCE. Simply ask the patient if they have noticed any change in their sense of smell lately. Ask if they can smell food, flowers etc. Formal smell identification and threshold tests exist, but are unlikely to be applicable to an OSCE situation.

Cranial nerve II – optic nerve

Acuity

Ideally this should be tested with a Snellen chart at six metres distance. If the patient usually wears glasses, they should keep them on. Test each eye separately, covering the other as appropriate. Invite the patient to read from the top line (largest letters) down as far as they can go. Record the findings as 6/6 if at six metres they can read down to line six, and 6/24 if at six metres they can read to line 24.

Colour

Formal assessment is made using Ishihara charts. Alternatively, you can ask about the colour of various objects in the room. Both eyes should be tested separately.

Fields

Start with screening for temporal field defects (isolated nasal field defects are exceptionally rare) and if you elicit any abnormalities, you can then perform confrontational testing on one eye at a time (for the OSCE, it is advisable to test the eyes individually, regardless of screening findings). It should be noted that any examination of visual fields by these methods is notoriously inaccurate. Any defects can be formally assessed using perimetry.

To screen for visual field defects, position yourself in front of the patient and ensure that your eyes are level with theirs. Ask them to focus on your nose and explain that you are going to move your fingers at what you think will be the boundaries of their visual field. Tell them to point at the finger that moves, whilst maintaining their gaze on your nose. Once they have understood and are gazing at your nose, raise both hands to the superior, outer quadrants of your visual field and test these one at a time. Repeat this for the inferior outer quadrants. You should ensure that your hands remain equidistant between the patient and yourself.

When one examines the field of each individual eye, it is necessary to assess all four quadrants. To do this, instruct the patient to cover one eye, and stare with their other eye into your corresponding eye (i.e. if the patient is covering their left eye, they should stare with their right eye directly into your left eye). Always start with your fingers at the extremes of the visual field, and move your finger in towards the centre. The patient should inform you as soon as they see the finger moving. Compare the patient's visual field to your own. Central, colour visual fields can also be tested using a red hat pin. Finally, the blind spot may be demonstrated by slowly bringing the hat pin in from a lateral position until the patient loses sight of it. This happens at about 30° from the midline, and it subsequently reappears medially. Blind spot mapping, if done, should also be performed in the vertical plane. Compare the blind spot to your own and note if it appears enlarged.

It is advisable to familiarise yourself with the most common visual field defects and how their presence localises to a specific area of the visual pathway.

Fundoscopy

It is important to mention this when examining CN II. However, in most cases it is examined as a separate OSCE station (*see* Chapter B5, Ophthalmoscopy).

Pupils

Begin with a simple inspection, commenting on their size and shape compared to each other. Ask the patient to look into the distance. Shine a bright pen torch at a short distance from one eye. Bring the pen torch in from a lateral position and observe for pupil constriction (the direct reflex). Bring the pen torch in again to the same eye from a lateral position and observe for constriction of the other pupil (the consensual reflex). Test each eye in turn. CN II is the afferent and CN III the efferent for the pupillary light reflex.

Examination for relative afferent pupillary defect (RAPD) should also be performed using the pen torch. A positive result confirms relative damage to the afferent nerve (CN II), compared to the other side. Shine the pen torch into one eye and observe bilateral pupil constriction. If one swings the light back and forth between the eyes, the pupils should continue to stay constricted. If, when the light is shone into the second eye, the pupils dilate, this is a positive result and confirms a defect of the afferent (CN II). The

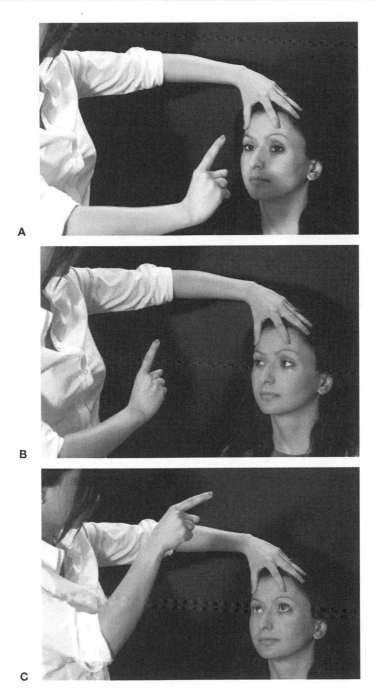

A

B

C

FIGURE A4.1 Testing extra-ocular movements

patient is said to have a RAPD. This finding may be supported by reduced visual acuity in the same eye, and indicates that disparity in acuity comes from optic nerve disease.

Demonstrate the accommodation reflex. Again, ask the patient to look into the distance. Bring your finger into the midline, approximately 10 cm from the patient's nose. Ask them to fix on your finger, and observe for convergence and pupil constriction.

Cranial nerves III, IV, VI – oculomotor, trochlear, abducens nerves

Ask the patient if they ever suffer from double vision, and if they do, what direction of gaze this occurs in. Lightly fix the patient's head and perform the 'H' test (*see* Figure A4.1). They should follow the finger with their eyes, and without moving their head. They should inform you if they develop double vision at any point. Observe for abnormalities in conjugate gaze whilst tracking, and also for nystagmus. Remember, it can be normal for nystagmus to occur at the extremes of lateral gaze.

Note the following:

- CN III supplies the medial rectus, inferior rectus, inferior oblique and superior rectus – look for a ptosis and also at the pupil; mydriasis occurs in surgical lesions of CN III
- CN IV supplies the superior oblique – if damaged, the head is often tilted away as compensation
- CN VI supplies the lateral rectus.

One can also test for saccadic eye movements, by asking the patient to look from side to side, and up and down.

Cranial nerve V – trigeminal nerve

Motor

Test the motor component of the nerve by asking the patient to clench their teeth whilst you feel the bulk of the masseter and temporalis muscles. Observe the jaw opening; if weak, it will deviate to the side of the lesion.

Perform the jaw jerk reflex by placing a finger below the lips of the patient, on the mandible, and lightly striking this with a tendon hammer. The patient should have their mouth slightly open. If positive, the jaw should jerk upwards.

Sensory

Test fine touch bilaterally in the areas of the face innervated by ophthalmic, maxillary and mandibular branches of the trigeminal nerve. You should touch in six places, three on each side, and compare sides as you do, using a piece of cotton wool. Ask the patient to tell you as you touch them, and if it feels the same as the other side. Stay close to the midline to ensure that you are not stimulating upper cervical nerve dermatomes at the angle of the mandible. Before starting, one should lightly touch the skin over sternum, since this central example helps the patient to understand what the sensation should feel like.

The corneal reflex tests CN V as the afferent and CN VII as the efferent. Ask the patient to look in a lateral direction and gently touch the cornea (not the conjunctiva) with a wisp of cotton. Observe for a blink reflex bilaterally.

Cranial nerve VII – facial nerve (see Figure A4.2)
Start by enquiring about the sense of taste, although it is unlikely that you will be able to test this formally. Inspect the face more thoroughly. Drooping of the corner of the mouth, loss of the nasolabial fold and absence of forehead wrinkling may indicate facial nerve damage.

Test the motor portion of the nerve by asking the patient to do the following:
- 'raise your eyebrows' – look for wrinkling of the forehead, which is preserved in upper motor neurone (UMN) facial nerve palsies and lost in lower motor neurone (LMN) palsies
- 'screw your eyes up, as if you have soap in them' – gently try to force them open, looking for burying of the eyelashes
- 'frown'
- 'puff your cheeks' – gently try to push the air out while they resist
- 'bare your teeth'.

Cranial nerve VIII – vestibulocochlear nerve
Occlude one ear whilst whispering a number quietly into the other ear. Ask the patient to repeat back what you have said. Alternatively, use the ticking of a mechanical watch to test this. These are gross screening tests but are adequate for the OSCE station if the patient reports no difference. If one does elicit a difference, then this should be further characterised as

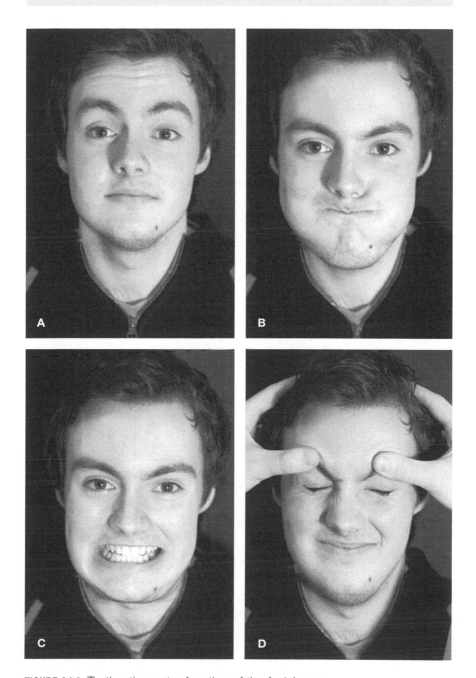

FIGURE A4.2 Testing the motor function of the facial nerve

to whether it is a conductive hearing problem or a sensorineural problem. This can be done using the Rinne and Weber tests.

Rinne test

Place a vibrating tuning fork (256 or 512 Hz) on the mastoid process, posterior to the ear. Ask the patient to tell you when they can no longer hear a sound. At that point, angle the fork towards the auricular meatus, the sound should be heard again. This is a normal test result, otherwise known as Rinne positive. Air conduction should be better than bone conduction. If sound is heard better through bone than through the normal conducting system (bone conduction is greater than air conduction), the patient has conductive hearing loss and is Rinne negative. In sensorineural deafness, air conduction often exceeds bone conduction, and so is Rinne positive, but may give false negatives. For this reason, the Rinne test should be used in conjunction with the Weber test.

Weber test

Place a vibrating tuning fork (256 or 512 Hz) on the centre of the forehead and ask the patient on which side the sound is best heard. In normal subjects, the sound should be heard in the centre of the head. If the sound lateralises, it means that they either have conductive deafness on that same side or sensorineural deafness on the other side.

Suspected hearing loss should be investigated further by an audiogram.

Cranial nerves IX, X – glossopharyngeal and vagus nerves

Ask the patient to open their mouth and say 'ahh'. Use a tongue depressor and a bright light to observe for symmetrical rising of the soft palate. If there is unilateral weakness, the uvula will deviate away from the weak side.

The gag reflex is rarely tested in an OSCE scenario. The afferent in the IXth, the efferent is the Xth.

Cranial nerve XI – accessory nerve

Ask the patient to rotate their head against resistance. Ask the patient to shrug their shoulders against resistance.

Cranial nerve XII – hypoglossal nerve

Observe the tongue at rest in the mouth. Look for deviation, atrophy and fasciculation. Ask the patient to stick out their tongue and observe for deviation. Test the strength as the patient pushes on the inside of their cheek with their tongue.

Completing your examination

Upon finishing your examination, thank the patient and ensure that they are comfortable. Wash your hands.

Comment that ideally, you would also examine the upper and lower extremities to further consolidate your findings.

Conclusion and presentation

Assimilate and present your findings, concentrating on the pertinent positives. Offer a diagnosis or a differential diagnosis.

An example of your presentation would be:

> This elderly gentleman has a right-sided facial weakness with sparing of the forehead, indicating an upper motor neuron lesion. He has a right homonymous hemianopia. He has a right hemifacial sensory loss and his uvula deviates to the left. In summary, this gentleman has signs consistent with a left-sided cortical lesion. Ideally, I would seek support for my diagnosis by performing an examination of the upper and lower extremities.

Example of a cranial nerve examination mark scheme

Before you start
- Makes introduction (full name and role)
- Offers explanation and seeks consent
- Ensures adequate exposure and patient's comfort
- Washes hands

Examination

General

- Makes general examination/inspection

The cranial nerves

- Mentions cranial nerve I
- Assesses visual acuity and colour vision
- Mentions fundoscopy
- Examines visual fields
- Makes appropriate examination of the pupils
- Tests the extra-ocular movements
- Tests motor and sensory components of cranial nerve V
- Offers to perform corneal reflex
- Tests facial movements
- Performs auditory screening, comments on Rinne and Weber tests
- Observes the palate, mentions the gag reflex
- Examines cranial nerve XI
- Examines the tongue
- Mentions further examination (peripheral neurological exam)

Completing your examination

- Ensures the patient is left comfortable
- Thanks patient
- Washes hands
- Demonstrates empathy
- Presents examination findings in a concise and confident manner
- Offers (differential) diagnosis
- Does the above in a fluent, professional manner

5

Peripheral neurological

Introduction

Neurological examinations have the tendency of unnerving students. Perhaps this is because we tend to use other examinations, such as the cardiovascular exam, more commonly and there is a lack of familiarity with the neurological exam. This should not be the case, and it is important to conduct at least a basic neurological examination on the majority of patients. In addition, students may be confused as to what exactly they are being asked to do. For example, it would be more appropriate to call the 'peripheral nervous system' examination 'a neurological examination of the extremities and trunk', since in it we are examining motor components (upper and lower motor neurones) and sensory components, not simply the peripheral nerves.

The neurological examination is frequently muddled, so this can be your chance to shine. Embark on the examination with a systematic approach, and there is little that you can do wrong. Due to time constraints in the examination, you are unlikely to be asked to examine both the upper and lower limbs, however, you must be prepared to do either, or both.

Before you start

Read the instructions carefully before you enter the station. Introduce yourself to the examiner and the patient. Briefly explain to the patient what you would like to do and gain verbal consent. Wash your hands and position yourself at the end of the bed. Ensure that the patient is lying comfortably and adequately exposed before starting the examination. It is worth asking the patient if they are left-handed or right-handed. However, they may not be allowed to tell you.

Examination
General
From the end of the bed, ask yourself:
- Does the patient look well or unwell?
- Are they comfortable at rest or in pain/distress?
- Is the patient adopting a specific posture (e.g. dystonic or flexed)?
- Do they have any abnormal movements/spontaneous movements (e.g. orofacial, tics, chorea, myoclonus)?
- Do they have any skin abnormalities (e.g. neurofibromas, rashes, herpes zoster, lipohypertrophy)?
- Are there paraphernalia around the bedside indicating an underlying illness, e.g. walking aids, wheelchair, shoes (callipers, built-up heels, scuffed toes), medications (including insulin pens), drug charts or neurological observation charts?

Inspection
Carefully inspect the upper/lower limbs for muscle wasting. When looking at the upper limbs, remember to look at the shoulders, and around the posterior aspect of the shoulder. When looking at the lower limbs, you also need to inspect the gluteal muscles. If you observe wasting, you should use a tape measure to quantify this.

Most of your inspection will have been completed from the end of the bed. However, on closer inspection look for the items listed above under *General*, plus:
- scars
- fasciculations
- tremors.

From this point, the examination will be separated into the upper limbs and the lower limbs.

The upper limbs

Drift

Ask the patient to stretch their arms out, with their palms facing upwards and their eyes closed. Observe for:

- pronator drift (the arm drops and pronates) – upper motor neurone lesions
- upward drift of the arms with oscillation – cerebellar disease
- pseudoathetosis of the fingers (the palms should be facing down for this) – sensory ataxia due to decreased joint position sense.

Tone

Ask the patient to fully relax whilst you passively move all major joints of the upper limb at random. The easiest way to do this is to take the patient by the hand, as though shaking hands, and roll the wrist, while flexing and extending the elbow, and rolling the shoulder. Tone can be:

- normal
- increased – described as spasticity or rigidity; causes for these include upper motor neurone lesions and extrapyramidal disease, respectively
- decreased – described as flaccidity; causes for this include lower motor neurone lesions and cerebellar disease.

Power

Power is traditionally graded on the Medical Research Council (MRC) scale of 0–5:

0 – no movement
1 – muscle flicker or minimal contraction
2 – active movement, with gravity eliminated
3 – active movement against gravity
4 – movement against gravity and resistance. This may be further divided into 4–, 4, 4+ to indicate movement against slight, moderate and strong resistance respectively
5 – normal power.

Test all movements in the upper limbs and ensure that you recognise the nerve roots and peripheral nerves that correlate with each movement. Ask your patient to perform the following movements while you assess their power:

43

- shoulder abduction – 'put your arms out to the side, like a chicken's wings, and don't let me push them down'
- shoulder adduction – 'bring your elbows back to your sides, while I try and prevent you'
- elbow flexion – 'put your arms up like a boxer, and don't let me straighten them'
- elbow extension – 'with your arms up like a boxer, push me away'
- wrist extension – 'cock your wrists back and don't let me straighten them'
- wrist flexion – 'make a fist, and push down against my hand'
- finger extension – 'straighten your hands out, palms down, and don't let me push your fingers down'
- finger abduction – 'splay your fingers out and don't let me push them back together'
- finger flexion – 'make a tight fist and don't let me straighten your fingers'
- finger adduction – place a piece of paper between the subject's fingers, asking 'squeeze the paper and don't let me pull it out'
- thumb abduction – 'with your palms facing up, point your thumb to the ceiling, and don't let me push it down'.

Reflexes

Practise eliciting reflexes to ensure that you know where the tendons lie anatomically. Hold the tendon hammer down the shaft, away from the head, and swing it purposefully. Reflexes can be described as:

- (pathologically) brisk (+++) – upper motor neurone lesions
- normal (++)
- reduced (+)
- absent (–)
- present only with reinforcement, i.e. teeth clenching (±).

When eliciting reflexes in the upper limb, you should gently lay the arm across the patient's body, with the elbow flexed to about 90°. Although there are other reflexes that can be tested, the following are essential when examining the upper limb:

- biceps reflex – C5/C6
- supinator reflex – C6
- triceps reflex – C7/C8.

Coordination

Coordination is often tested last when assessing motor function. This is because weakness can cause features that appear similar to reduced coordination.

Finger–nose testing

Raise your index finger at one arm's length from the patient. Ask the patient to extend their index finger and touch your finger and then touch their nose. Their arm should be fully extended when their finger meets yours. Guide them physically for the first few journeys. The pulp of the patient's fingertip should make contact with both your finger and their nose, and therefore must rotate through 180°. Ask the patient to repeat this movement as accurately as possible. Look for action and intention tremors, and the rate and range of movement. Compare both sides. If you wish to assess cerebellar signs, move your index finger slightly closer to the patient to assess for past-pointing.

Dysdiadochokinesis

This is the failure to perform alternating movements. Ask the patient to tap the palm and the dorsum of the hand alternately on the palm of the other hand. It is normal for the non-dominant hand to be a little less coordinated.

Joint position sensation

Joint position sensation (JPS) tests proprioceptive function and the relevant fibres project through the dorsal columns. Take the patient's hand, holding the lateral borders of the index finger between the distal interphalangeal (DIP) joint and the proximal interphalangeal (PIP) joint. Move the distal phalanx up and down, explaining to the patient which direction is which. Be sure to only touch the lateral borders of the distal phalanx to eliminate pressure sensation on the nail bed.

Ask the patient to close their eyes and tell you which direction you are moving the joint. Start initially with small movements, increasing the size of movement if they are not able to detect it initially. If they are unable to detect movement distally, move to the next joint, working proximally until they are able to tell you the direction of joint movement.

Vibration sensation

Vibration sense is carried within the dorsal columns, and should be tested using a 128-Hz tuning fork. Start by testing the tuning fork on the sternum to ensure that the patient is able to feel the vibration.

Starting distally, place the vibrating tuning fork on the DIP joint and ask the patient if they are able to feel the vibration. Ask the patient to close their eyes and inform you when the vibration stops. Stop the vibration suddenly by holding the distal end of the tuning fork. If the patient is unable to feel the vibration or to tell you when it stops, move proximally to the next bony prominence, the PIP, the metacarpophalangeal joint (MCP), and then onto the ulnar styloid, until the patient is able to sense the vibration.

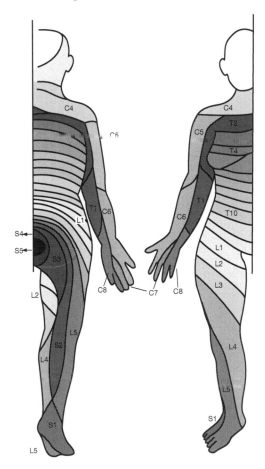

FIGURE A5.1 Dermatomes

Touch sensation

You should test both pin-prick and fine touch:

- fine touch (dorsal columns)
- pin-prick (spinothalamic tract).

Test fine touch using a wisp of cotton wool. Start by ensuring that the patient can feel the wisp of cotton wool on the sternum. Ask the patient to close their eyes, and test all dermatomes of the upper limbs (*see* Figure A5.1). Ask the patient to say 'yes' every time they feel you touch them. Ensure that there is no variation between the two sides. When touching the patient with the cotton wool, be sure to use a dabbing motion and never a stroking motion. Stroking will result in a tickle sensation that also projects through the spinothalamic pathway.

Map out any sensory deficits as you go, asking yourself:

- Does this fit a dermatomal/peripheral nerve distribution?
- Is this a distal sensory deficit (e.g. glove distribution)?

Test pin-prick using a single-use neurological examination pin, and follow the same process used for fine touch. Never use a needle.

The lower limbs

Examination of the lower limbs follows a very similar format to that of the upper limbs. However, there are a few variations.

Gait

Start by asking the patient to walk for several metres, then turn and walk back towards you. If you feel that they may be unsteady or likely to fall, ask the examiner or a nurse to assist the patient and walk alongside them.

Observe for the following:

- transfer from the chair or bed to the standing position
- stride length and regularity
- ataxia
- arm swinging
- posture
- involuntary movements.

Ask the patient to stand in front of you and perform the following:
- stand on their toes – tests for weakness of the gastrocnemius and soleus muscles
- stand on their heels – demonstrates foot drop.

Before sitting the patient down, perform Romberg's test.
- This test is to assess joint position sense.
- Ask the patient to stand with their feet together and their eyes open. Check that they are steady and then ask them to close their eyes. If they are unsteady with their eyes open, the test should stop before eye closure.
- Romberg's is only positive in those who start to fall before you prevent them once their eyes are closed. Poor balance can cause increased sway, but is not a positive Romberg's test.

Tone

The remainder of the examination can be conducted with the patient reclined on the couch. Explain to the patient that they must relax as much as possible, then:
- one at a time, roll the legs from side to side, making an assessment of tone
- suddenly lift the leg from behind the knee – the foot should not ordinarily leave the bed; increased tone is indicated if the foot does leave the bed
- test for ankle clonus – more than five beats of clonus are described as sustained.

Power

As with the upper limbs, power is graded 0–5. Ensure that you test each individual movement, noting abnormalities as you go. Ask your patient to perform the following movements whilst you apply resistance:
- hip extension – 'lift your leg straight up off the bed and don't let me push it back down'
- hip flexion – 'push your leg down into the bed and don't let me lift it up off'
- hip abduction – 'open your legs, while I try to stop you'
- hip adduction – 'close your legs, while I try to stop you'

- knee flexion – 'bend your knee and don't let me straighten it out'
- knee extension – 'with your knee from the bent position, kick me away and straighten your leg'
- ankle dorsiflexion – 'point your toes towards your head and don't let me pull them down'
- ankle plantarflexion – 'push your feet down against my hands, as if trying to stand on your toes.'

Reflexes

Using the same grading as described for the upper limbs, test the following reflexes:

- ankle reflex – S1/S2
- patellar reflex – L3/L4
- plantar reflex – using an orange stick, gently scratch the lateral edge of the sole from the heel to the 5th toe, and then medially along the metatarsal heads. The normal response is down-going plantars. An extensor (up-going) response, so-called Babinski's sign, is indicative of upper motor neurone pathology. Always warn the patient before you test their plantars, as it is often uncomfortable.

Coordination

Assess coordination with the heel–shin test. With the patient's eyes open, ask them to run the heel of one foot down their shin on the other side, from the knee to the foot. Make a comparison of both sides. It can be difficult to assess coordination if there is lower limb weakness.

Joint position sensation

Start distally at the toes, and move proximally until the patient is able to correctly sense the direction of movement. Ensure that you show the patient which way is up and which is down when their eyes are open, before asking them to close their eyes to assess their JPS.

Vibration sensation

Again, begin on the most distal joint of the great toe, and gradually work more proximally if vibration sensation is not felt. If the patient detects the vibration, ask them to tell you when it stops before deadening the tuning fork with your fingers.

Touch sensation

Ensure that you are familiar with the dermatomes and also the cutaneous distribution of peripheral nerves. Attempt to map out any abnormalities in sensation. Test both fine touch and pin-prick sensation.

Completing your examination

Having completed your examination, you should cover the patient and thank them. Ensure that they are comfortable. Wash your hands.

One can comment on the wish to undertake an examination of the cranial nerves, if appropriate. It may be unwise in a neurological examination to signal to the examiner any further investigations (such as imaging or neurophysiology) that you would like to request, unless you are asked to do so. The indications for these investigations are quite specific and you may dig yourself into a hole having conducted a good practical examination.

Conclusion and presentation

Spend a few moments gathering your thoughts prior to presenting your findings and summary to the examiner. Present your findings in a logical, systematic way, reporting on both the pertinent negatives and positives from your examination. Try to offer a diagnosis or differential diagnosis.

An example of a confident presentation may be:

> This right-hand-dominant, 79-year-old gentleman appears to be comfortable at rest, however, his left arm is held in a flexed posture, consistent with a left hemiparesis, and this is apparent from the end of the bed. There does not appear to be any obvious muscle wasting. There are no fasciculations, scars or skin changes. The right side appears normal on inspection.
>
> There is markedly increased tone in the left arm and leg, and power is reduced at 2/5 in all movements of the left lower limb, and 3/5 in all movements of the left upper limb. Reflexes are pathologically brisk on the left, accompanied by an up-going left plantar reflex and down-going right. It was not possible to assess coordination in the left arm or leg, due to weakness. Sensation is decreased in all modalities on the left. Tone, power, reflexes, coordination and all sensory modalities appear normal in the right upper and lower limbs. As a result of weakness, the patient is unable to get out of bed, and I therefore feel that it is unsafe to try to assess gait and Romberg's test.

There is a wheelchair at the bedside, and I note that there is also an insulin pen, together with a blood glucose monitoring chart.

The findings are consistent with a right middle cerebral artery territory stroke, resulting in a dense left hemiparesis. I would like to further examine this patient by conducting a swallowing assessment and cranial nerves examination.

Example of a peripheral nervous system examination mark scheme

Before you start
- Makes introduction (full name and role)
- Offers explanation and seeks consent
- Ensures adequate exposure and patient's comfort
- Washes hands

Examination
General
- Comments on general appearance

Inspection
- Notes any important neurological features on inspection

The upper limbs and the lower limbs
- Makes a correct assessment of tone
- Makes a correct assessment of power
- Correctly elicits reflexes (in the event of an absent reflex, repeats reflex testing with re-enforcement manoeuvres)
- Checks plantar response and is able to correctly interpret
- Assesses co-ordination correctly and understands the limitations of patients with decreased power
- Assesses joint position sensation
- Assesses vibration sensation

- Assesses fine touch and pin-prick sensation
- Mentions further examination (e.g. cranial nerves exam)

Completing your examination
- Covers the patient, ensuring that they are comfortable
- Thanks patient
- Washes hands
- Demonstrates empathy
- Presents examination findings in a concise and confident manner
- Offers (differential) diagnosis
- Does the above in a fluent, professional manner

6

Lumps and bumps

Introduction

The finding of a lump is a common reason for patients to present to their medical practitioner. Some lumps are also found on routine examination. No matter what the anatomical location, the process of examining a lump remains consistent. It is necessary to determine the diagnosis of a lump and what sort of treatment, if any, may be offered.

Before you start

Enter the station and read the instructions. Introduce yourself to both the patient and examiner. Gain verbal consent from the patient to examine the lump. You will need to expose the area around the lump, and also the regional lymphatics that drain the area. In some instances, it may be appropriate to have a chaperone present e.g. breast or groin lumps. Ensure that the patient is comfortable, and wash your hands.

Examination

General

Standing at the end of the bed, look at the patient and ask yourself the following:

- Does the patient look well or unwell?
- Are they in obvious pain/discomfort?
- Can you see the lump from the end of the bed?

- Are there paraphernalia around the bed indicating why the patient is in hospital?

Inspection

If the lump is not immediately apparent, ask the patient to indicate where they felt the lump. Inspect the lump, noting:
- its anatomical location
- skin colour changes
- skin texture changes
- other obvious abnormalities, such as sinus tracts etc.
- its size
- if the edges are well defined
- if it is visibly pulsatile.

Palpation

A large amount of information will be gained through palpation. Before doing so, ask the patient if it is painful or tender to touch. If they report it to be painful, explain that you will need to feel the area and that if it is too uncomfortable they should inform you and you will stop. Consider the following during palpation:
- temperature – compared to surrounding tissue
- tenderness
- size – use a measuring tape; this is especially important to repeat in the future to see if the mass is changing in size
- position – sometimes the origin of a mass is obvious – e.g. thyroid or breast – but it is often less clear in areas such as the abdomen
- attachments – a mass may fix itself to surrounding structures. This may be the skin, subcutaneous tissue, muscle, arteries, veins or deeper structures. Attachment to blood vessels may cause masses to become pulsatile or have a palpable thrill. Attachment to underlying muscle can be ascertained by asking the patient to tense the muscles in the area of the mass to see if a previously mobile mass becomes immobile
- surface – this can either be smooth or irregular, and may provide clues to the underlying pathological process – e.g. when palpating the liver, a hard, irregular liver edge could signify malignancy, while a smooth, tender liver edge could signify an acute hepatitis

- margin – can the borders of the mass easily be defined? Are the borders of the mass regular or irregular, sharp or rounded?
- consistency – may give clues as to the diagnosis; hard masses may be malignant or calcified, while soft, fluctuant masses tend to be fluid filled (abscess or cyst)
- transillumination – in a darkened room, press the lighted end of a pen torch into the side of the lump. If the lump lights up, this indicates a cystic swelling full of fluid
- thrills, pulsatility and bruits – if the mass is highly vascularised or vascular in origin, it may be pulsatile. There may also be a palpable thrill or you may hear a bruit with your stethoscope
- reducibility – can you reduce the mass by continued pressure? If so, this may indicate a hernia.

Depending upon your findings, it may also be appropriate to examine the lymph nodes that drain the region in which the lump is located. For example, if a breast lump is found, you should also examine the axillary lymph nodes.

Percussion
It is not always appropriate to percuss a mass, however, if the mass appears to be in the right upper quadrant of the abdomen, consistent with the liver, you must define the borders by percussion. Note if the mass is dull or resonant to percussion.

Auscultation
Suspicion of a hernia or vascular mass should prompt auscultation. Some examples of masses with important findings on auscultation are:
- arteriovenous malformations, arteriovenous fistulae (for renal dialysis) – systolic bruit
- hernia – bowel sounds indicating intestinal contents.

The hernia examination
To conduct a hernia examination in full, the patient should be examined in both standing and lying positions. A strong understanding of anatomy will aid diagnosis.

Many hernias will spontaneously reduce when the patient lies supine. Start with the patient standing and then:

- closely inspect the areas of the inguinal and femoral canals, and the scrotum in males, for any lumps or swellings
- ask the patient if they have any pain or tenderness
- ask the patient to cough and observe/palpate for a cough impulse
- using anatomical landmarks, identify the location of the lump relative to the pubic tubercle and inguinal ligament. This enables distinction between femoral and inguinal hernias
- to further identify the origin of the hernia, gauge the relationship of the lump to the femoral canal, and the internal and external inguinal rings
- ask the patient to lie flat, to see if the hernia reduces spontaneously
- if the hernia does not spontaneously reduce, try to reduce the lump yourself
- in the reduced hernia, assess for the cough impulse by pressing over the internal inguinal ring (mid-inguinal point) and ask the patient to cough
- maintain pressure over the internal inguinal ring while asking the patient to stand – if you can prevent it from re-appearing, it is an indirect inguinal hernia
- be sure to examine the normal side.

Completing your examination

Remember to examine the lymph nodes local to the mass, if you have not already done so (*see* above). Cover the patient and ensure that they are comfortable. Thank the patient. Wash your hands.

Once you have completed your examination, you may wish to mention further investigations, such as imaging followed by biopsy or aspiration (if appropriate).

Conclusion and presentation

Spend a few moments gathering and organising your thoughts before presenting your findings to the examiner. Offer a diagnosis or differential diagnosis.

An example of your presentation may be:

This is a 38-year-old lady who looks well and comfortable at rest. There is a mass over the anterior aspect of the left forearm with an overlying well-healed scar. The mass is non-tender and measures 9 cm by 2 cm. There are no changes to the surrounding skin or temperature differences, and the skin is freely mobile over the surface. It does not appear to be attached to the underlying muscle. The mass is soft but does not transilluminate. I can palpate a thrill, and auscultate a bruit. These findings are consistent with a left forearm arterio-venous fistula.

Example of a lumps and bumps examination mark scheme

Before you start
- Makes introduction (full name and role)
- Offers explanation and seeks consent
- Offers chaperone (where appropriate)
- Ensures adequate exposure and patient's comfort
- Positions patient appropriately
- Washes hands

Examination
- Comments on general appearance
- Makes detailed inspection of the lump
- Checks for pain
- Correctly palpates the lump
- Describes the lump fully
- Examines local lymph nodes
- Conducts a hernia examination correctly, if appropriate

Completing your examination
- Covers the patient, ensuring that they are comfortable
- Thanks patient
- Washes hands

- Demonstrates empathy
- Presents examination findings in a concise and confident manner
- Offers (differential) diagnosis
- Does the above in a fluent, professional manner

7

Breast

Introduction

This is easily the most terrifying clinical examination that you are required to perform in the final OSCE. It is made additionally awkward by the fact that the patient is often female with a large pair of 'pretend' breasts strapped to her chest. It is important not to let that put you off and to maintain a professional attitude. Breast examinations are often frightening for the patient as well. It is important that you put them at ease, since a tense patient, particularly in 'real' situations, will be difficult to examine.

The best possible way to prepare for this examination is to ensure that you have done it in real life. You should take an opportunity to attend a breast clinic during your clinical training.

It is important to recognise that clinical examination forms part of the triple assessment of breast disease. In almost all cases, discovery of a lump will be followed up with mammography and/or ultrasonography, depending on the patient's age (mammogram is not recommended for those under 35 years). Following this, fine needle aspiration for cytology (FNAC) or core biopsy may be used to gain tissue for diagnosis.

Before you start

Enter the station and read your instructions carefully, since the station may ask you to examine only one breast. The station may well combine the aspects of breast examination with those of examining and describing a lump (see Chapter A6, Lumps and bumps). Introduce yourself to the patient and the examiner. There should be a female chaperone present at all times and the patient should be wearing a front-tying gown. Explain to the patient what you wish to do, why it is necessary, and gain their consent to proceed. Wash your hands thoroughly.

Ask the patient if they regularly self-examine, and if they have found any lumps during this. If yes, ask them to point to where they have found it/them.

You will need to see the patient in a number of positions during this examination, but it is probably best to start with them perched on the edge of the couch with their legs dangling. Once ready, reassure the patient and ask them to lower the gown. You should turn away whilst they uncover the upper part of their body.

Examination
General
Stand in front of the patient, who should be sat upright, comfortably, with breasts exposed and arms at rest by their sides. Ask yourself:
- Does the patient look well or unwell?
- Is the patient comfortable or are they in pain/distress?

Inspection (see Figure A7.1)
Paying reference to the breasts themselves, look for any:
- asymmetry – general or localised (i.e. an obvious mass)
- signs of inflammation – redness or oedema, which often resembles the skin of an orange (*peau d'orange*)
- nipple inversion or eczema around the nipple
- blood or discharge from the nipple
- tethering or dimpling of the skin
- surgical scars – check beneath, around the areola, in the axilla.

Now ask the patient to put their hands behind their head and push their elbows back, so they are in line with the shoulders. Observe for the above again. Finally, ask them to place their hands on their waist and push forcibly inwards. This contracts the pectoralis major muscle and may emphasise any tethering that is present. Repeat your observations in this position.

An optional extra is to ask the patient to lean forwards, to allow the

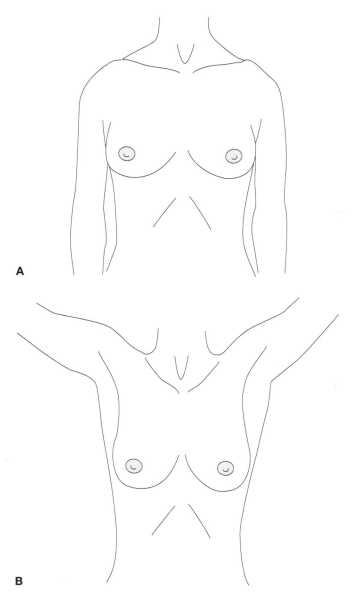

A

B

FIGURE A7.1 Positions for inspection of the breasts

breasts to hang down, which may once again emphasise any abnormalities. Otherwise, at this point, ask the patient to lie semi-recumbent on the couch, with a cushion or pillow under the shoulders, for the remainder of the examination.

Palpation

Ask the patient if they have any breast pain and, if yes, whereabouts the pain is. You should use the flat of your hand when you examine the breast and only use tips of the fingers to explore a lump.

If the patient has indicated that they have found a lump in one of their breasts, start your examination on the normal side. There are two main techniques for breast examination, although you may have seen clinicians perform variations of these. You can use a 'lawnmower' technique, starting in one corner of the examination field and palpating from side to side or up and down systematically until you have covered the entire breast, including the axillary tail. Alternatively, one can divide the breast into quarters (plus the central nipple area) and palpate each of these five areas separately.

If you discover a lump whilst palpating, it is important to further characterise it according to the following features:

- size
- shape
- site
- surface
- colour of overlying skin
- temperature of overlying skin
- mobility
- attachments
- fluctuance.

Remember that there may well be more than one lump in a breast, so continue to examine even after you are satisfied with your assessment of the first lump. Pass comment on any lumps present and the number palpated. Once you have completed examining the first breast, palpation should continue with comparison to the other breast.

It is important to examine for lymphadenopathy in the axillae and supraclavicularly. When examining the axilla, ask the patient to allow you to take the full weight of the ipsilateral arm. Gently push your fingertips into the axilla, feeling medially, laterally and apically for any palpable lymph nodes. Repeat both sides. You may need to ask the patient to sit up to examine the axillary lymph nodes adequately.

Some clinicians recline the patient further and examine for an enlarged liver, and also may sit the patient forward and examine for spinal tenderness, or examine the chest. This is usually done when metastatic disease is suspected, or needs to be excluded.

Completing your examination

There is nothing on the breast examination to percuss or auscultate, unless you are excluding liver or lung metastases, so once you have finished palpating, cover the patient and thank them. Wash your hands.

Conclusion and presentation

Gather your thoughts before presenting your findings to the examiner. Present your findings systematically and offer a diagnosis. For example:

> This 45-year-old lady has a 2 cm by 3 cm irregular lump in the upper, outer quadrant of her right breast. The overlying skin is dimpled and this is exaggerated with contraction of pectoralis major. The lump itself has limited mobility and appears to be attached to the underlying muscle and indeed to the overlying skin. There is no nipple involvement, however, there is ipsilateral axillary lymphadenopathy with three nodes individually palpable. There are no abnormalities on the left. In light of these findings, I would suggest that this lady most likely has a breast malignancy and will need radiographic imaging, with or without ultrasonography, and tissue sampling to confirm the diagnosis.

A conclusion such as the above will help a candidate to score highly, because it bridges the gap between clinical examination skills and their application to clinical medicine. This is the endpoint goal for all of us; using our examination skills to make clinical diagnoses and plan further investigation and treatment. The really confident/experienced candidate may wish to give the examination findings a 'P' value (clinical findings on palpation):

P1   normal breast tissue, no lumps or nodularities
P2   benign changes, nodularities or lump with benign features, e.g. smooth, well demarcated, firm and easily movable
P3   abnormal but likely to be benign
P4   suspicious lump

P5   malignant, with all features of a malignant lump, e.g. hard, irregular, fixed to skin or underlying muscle.

Example of a breast examination mark scheme

Before you start
- Makes introduction (full name and role)
- Offers explanation and seeks consent
- Offers chaperone
- Ensures adequate exposure and patient's comfort
- Positions patient appropriately for each examination stage
- Washes hands

Examination
- Makes inspection (commenting on asymmetry, dimpling, nipple inversion, discharge)
- Palpates all breast areas using recognised technique
- Identifies breast lump and its features
- Describes breast lump
- Palpates the axillae (supraclavicular fossa) for lymphadenopathy

Completing your examination
- Covers the patient, ensuring that they are comfortable
- Thanks patient
- Washes hands
- Demonstrates empathy
- Presents examination findings in a concise and confident manner
- Offers (differential) diagnosis
- Does the above in a fluent, professional manner

8

Thyroid/neck

Introduction

Examination of the neck may arise in two contexts. The first is examination of the thyroid gland and peripheral manifestations of thyroid disease. The other is the examination of a lump, describing it and formulating a differential diagnosis.

Examination of any lump is described elsewhere in this book (*see* Chapter A6, Lumps and bumps). However, it is useful to list some of the possible lumps that may arise in the neck. The sternocleidomastoid muscle is used to divide the neck into anterior and posterior triangles.

Anterior triangle lumps:
- thyroid gland (nodule, carcinoma, goitre)
- thyroglossal cyst
- lymph node
- pharyngeal pouch
- branchial cyst
- carotid body tumour
- keloid scar.

Posterior triangle lumps:
- lymph node
- cervical rib
- cystic hygroma
- subclavian artery aneurysm
- keloid scar.

Before you start

Enter the station, read the instructions and introduce yourself to the patient and the examiner. To reiterate, the examination will either be a general neck examination in which there will be a lump to find, or a scenario that encourages you to look for thyroid disease. We will cover the latter scenario in detail here.

You will need some equipment for this examination, so ensure that you have a glass of water and a tendon hammer at your disposal. Ideally, the patient should be perched on the edge of the couch or sat in a chair, so you can walk behind them to examine the neck. The patient should be adequately exposed, so that the whole of their neck and the upper part of their sternum can be seen. Explain to the patient what you wish to do, and why it is necessary. Gain their verbal consent to proceed. Wash your hands.

Examination

General

Standing in front of the patient, ask yourself:
- Does the patient look well or unwell?
- Are they comfortable at rest or are they in any pain/distress?
- Are they thin or overweight?
- Are they dressed appropriately for the ambient temperature?
- Do they have eye signs consistent with thyroid disease?
- Are they fidgety/restless or apathetic with myxoedematous facies?
- Are there any visible lumps?

The clinical examination is easier if you follow the standard inspection, palpation, percussion, auscultation process used for other system examinations.

The hands

Start at the hands and look for:
- palmar erythema (a hyperdynamic circulation occurs in thyrotoxicosis)
- tremor (occurs in thyrotoxicosis) – can be exaggerated by asking the patient to stretch out their hands together, with wrists in a neutral position, and elbows extended. Place a piece of paper on the back of the hands to emphasise very fine/low amplitude tremors (*see* Figure A8.1)

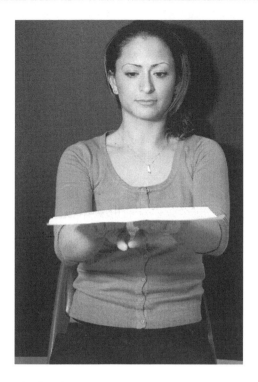

FIGURE A8.1 Demonstrating tremor

- acropachy – characteristically appears like clubbing and associated specifically with Graves' disease
- skin and temperature – warm and sweaty would suggest thyrotoxicity, whereas coarse and dry would suggest hypothyroidism.

Palpate the pulse. Abnormalities in rate may occur in thyroid disease (bradycardia in hypothyroidism, tachycardia in hyperthyroidism), as well as abnormalities in rhythm (atrial fibrillation in hyperthyroidism).

The eyes

Look at the eyes. Graves' disease is characterised by eye signs in the context of hyperthyroidism, but eye signs may also occur after treatment for this (when euthyroid or hypothyroid). Look for:

- proptosis – forward protrusion of an eye
- exophthalmos – with the eyes looking forward and relaxed, the upper and lower eyelids normally obscure the upper and lower rims of the

iris and the sclera above and below it. If exophthalmos is present, white sclera is observed above the lower lid
- lid retraction – sclera visible above the cornea
- chemosis – injection and oedema of the conjunctiva
- extra-ocular movement impairment, leading to diplopia.

Complete the eye examination by checking for lid-lag. Comment on loss of hair from the eyebrows.

The thyroid/neck

Inspection

Inspection of the neck involves the following:
- look for a goitre or other swelling in the region of the thyroid gland and comment if you find a mass
- ask the patient to swallow some water – if the identified mass is the thyroid gland or thyroglossal cyst, it will move
- ask the patient to protrude their tongue – if the lump is a thyroglossal cyst, it will move, but if it is the thyroid gland, it will stay still.

Make a final check for any surgical scars and then proceed to palpation.

Palpation (see Figure A8.2)

Move round the couch/chair to stand behind the patient. Explain to them that this is important in order to perform the examination properly. The examination may be uncomfortable but should not painful (unless they have thyroiditis). As a result, you must ask the patient if they have any pain before palpating. Warm your hands, since cold hands may make it difficult for the patient to relax the neck adequately for examination.

Place your hands gently on the patient's neck, again warning them before you do so. Identify the thyroid gland and palpate fully. Identify:
- Its borders (including feeling in the suprastrenal notch for retrosternal extension)
- the two lobes, the pyramid and the isthmus
- focal swelling/nodule
- diffuse enlargement
- tenderness
- its consistency.

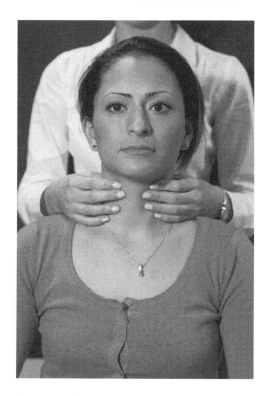

FIGURE A8.2 Palpation of the thyroid gland

Once you have identified a lump, ask the patient to assist your examination by taking a sip of water in the mouth, and then, while you are looking at the neck, ask them to swallow again. Some people gently push the thyroid to one side to enable improved palpation of one lobe at a time. Once you are satisfied that you can describe the gland as you would any other lump (*see* Chapter A6, Lumps and bumps), continue to palpate the remainder of the neck. Palpate specifically for any lymphadenopathy (supraclavicular, submandibular, postauricular and suboccipital).

Percussion and auscultation
If the thyroid is found to be enlarged, and you could not feel below the lower poles of the thyroid, percuss down the sternum to illustrate whether the thyroid extends retrosternally. You should examine to ensure that the trachea is central and not compromised.

An enlarged thyroid gland in Graves' disease may produce a bruit on auscultation of each lobe. You should put the stethoscope over the area of the superior thyroid artery.

Completing the examination

Expose the patient's shins and look for pretibial myxoedema (specific to Graves' disease). Ask the patient to rise from a seated position, without using their hands, to check for proximal myopathy. Check the ankle reflexes with a tendon hammer to discover whether they are brisk or slow-relaxing.

Cover the patient adequately, if they were exposed for any reason, and ensure their comfort. Thank the patient. Wash your hands and take a moment to gather your thoughts.

Conclusion and presentation

Summarise your findings to the examiner in a concise manner, drawing on the significant positive findings and any important negatives. Offer a diagnosis. For example:

> This middle-aged lady has a low body mass index, a fine tremor and a regular tachycardia at rest. She has exophthalmos and discernible lid-lag. Her thyroid gland is diffusely enlarged, however, the right lobe is greater in size than the left. The thyroid does not extend retrosternally, but has an audible bruit. She has no regional lymphadenopathy and no pretibial myxoedema. Her tendon reflexes are brisk. In light of these findings, I believe that this lady has hyperthyroidism due to Graves' disease and, as such, requires thyroid function testing and a thyroid antibody screen.

Example of a thyroid examination mark scheme

Before you start
- Makes introduction (full name and role)
- Offers explanation and seeks consent
- Ensures adequate exposure and patient's comfort

- Positions patient appropriately for each examination stage
- Washes hands

Examination

- Makes general inspection (including hands and pulse)
- Makes inspection of neck (comments on neck, watches patient swallowing)
- Makes inspection of eyes
- Palpates (from behind the patient)
- Percusses retrosternally
- Auscultates for bruits
- Examines legs

Completing your examination

- Covers the patient, ensuring that they are comfortable
- Thanks patient
- Washes hands
- Demonstrates empathy
- Presents examination findings in a concise and confident manner
- Offers (differential) diagnosis
- Does the above in a fluent, professional manner

9

Vascular

Introduction

There are always plenty of patients in hospital with either arterial or venous disease. Make sure that you recognise the different clinical examination features of both types of patient. Remember that many patients will have a combination of both arterial and venous disease. Ensure that you are familiar with the vascular anatomy of the lower limbs. Without this knowledge, interpretation of your findings and diagnosis is difficult.

There are key words that you must be familiar with when describing ulcerated lesions. If you state that an ulcer has a punched-out appearance, you are implying that it is an arterial ulcer. As such, be cautious of the descriptions you use. It is unlikely that you will be asked to conduct both arterial and venous examinations of the lower limbs.

Before you start

Read the instructions carefully and enter the station. Introduce yourself to the patient and the examiner. Gain verbal consent to perform the examination, by explaining what it will involve. Wash your hands and position yourself at the end of the bed. Ensure that the patient is comfortable and adequately exposed.

Examination

General

This should be conducted from the end of the bed. Ask yourself:

- Does the patient look well or unwell?
- Are there mobility aids around the bedside?
- Are there paraphernalia around the bedside indicating the underlying pathology, e.g. medications (insulin/oral hypoglycaemic agents), disease-monitoring equipment (glucometers)?

Take this opportunity to ask the patient if they have any pain.

Inspection

With the patient lying on the bed, inspect the legs carefully. Always compare sides.

- Are there any amputated limbs or toes?
- Is there evidence of muscle wasting?
- Is there any hair loss?
- Is there evidence of trophic skin change – e.g. colour changes? Look for eczematous changes, haemosiderin staining, lipodermatosclerosis, and dilated superficial veins. Comment on the distribution of any findings.
- Are there any scars? Ensure that you externally rotate the legs to look for scars medially. Look closely for stab incision marks from varicose vein surgery, and inspect the groins for scars from angiogram wires.
- Look for pulsatile masses.
- Inspect the legs for ulcerative lesions, ensuring that you look between the toe webs.

Describe any lesions that you observe, stating their location, size and characteristics.

Venous ulcers look completely different to arterial ulcers. The features listed in the table are meant to be a guide. They are not hard rules.

Palpation

Comparing both sides, feel the legs with the dorsum of your hand and comment on the temperature of the legs.

Palpate the legs for areas of tenderness, particularly the calf areas if you suspect deep vein thrombosis (DVT).

	VENOUS	ARTERIAL
Gender	Female	Male
Age	40–50 years	>60 years
Risk factors	Family history, previous DVT, pregnancy	Smoking, diabetes, hypercholesterolaemia, hypertension
Pain	More commonly with occlusive thrombosis	Severe pain, unless the patient has diabetic neuropathy
Site	Gaiter distribution	Pressure areas
Border	Irregular, erythematous edges	Well-circumscribed margin with punched-out appearance
Base	Pink and granulating	Sloughy (green) or necrotic (black)
Surrounding skin	Erythematous, haemosiderin staining, lipodermatosclerosis	Pale unless infected

Check the capillary refill time of both legs. Count for 5 seconds whilst gently squeezing the nail bed of the great toe. Release it, and count the number of seconds taken for colour to return (count out loud). It is normal for capillary refill to take up to 2 seconds.

Venous examination (additional points)
Venous disease is far more common in the lower limbs than in the upper limbs. It will usually present in one of four ways:
- varicose veins
- DVT
- superficial thrombosis/thrombophlebitis
- ulceration or trophic skin changes secondary to chronic venous insufficiency.

Inspection
The venous system can only be properly assessed with the patient standing.
Inspect the following:
- varicose veins (dilated superficial tortuous veins) – comment on the distribution of the varicosities. Remember that the long saphenous vein runs medially up to the level of the groin, and the short saphenous vein runs laterally up to the level of the knee
- other venous disease – i.e. DVT (redness, pain and swelling).

Varicose veins

Both the cough and tap tests for varicose veins are outdated and will tell you very little. The Trendelenburg test is also outdated, largely having been replaced by Doppler and Duplex scanning. However, it is worth knowing about it for your examination.

The Trendelenburg test is used to assess the pattern of venous incompetence in the leg.

- Lie the patient down, and elevate the leg to about 15° above horizontal to empty the superficial veins. This may be helped by 'milking' the leg. Note venous guttering.
- With the patient's leg still elevated, press with your thumb (or apply a tourniquet) over the saphenofemoral junction (SFJ). This is located 2–3 cm below and 2–3 cm lateral to the pubic tubercle.
- Ask the patient to stand while you maintain pressure over the SFJ.
- If the veins do not fill, this indicates SFJ incompetence. Releasing the pressure over the SFJ will confirm this if the veins subsequently fill up.

Arterial examination (additional points)

The general inspection and palpation will cover the majority of the initial part of the examination. Make sure that you comment on any amputations, scars or ulcerated lesions (*see* above).

Palpation of arterial pulses

Having compared the temperature of both legs, you must feel for all of the peripheral pulses. Use a system and either work proximal to distal, or vice versa. Ensure that the following pulses are palpated during your examination:

- abdominal aorta – palpate for an expansile, pulsatile mass consistent with an abdominal aortic aneurysm
- femoral
- popliteal
- posterior tibial
- dorsalis pedis (this may be absent in 10–15% of the population as a normal variant).

Note any absent or aneurismal pulses.

A sensory examination should also be conducted. In diabetic patients, you may well find a glove and stocking distribution of sensory deficit. In patients who present with a history consistent with an acute arterial occlusion, loss of sensation is one of the indications for urgent intervention.

Buerger's test

While the patient is laying flat on the couch, elevate their leg to 45° above the horizontal (*see* Figure A9.1). Support the patient's leg in this position for 2–3 minutes.

Ask the patient to sit up and swing their legs over the edge of the bed. Look at the patient's leg for 2–3 minutes. Buerger's test is positive if the patient's legs turn a waxy, cadaveric white colour on elevation with empty-ing, or 'guttering' of the superficial veins, followed by a reactive hyperaemia on dependency. This implies significant arterial insufficiency.

Completing your examination

Once you have conducted your examination, and depending on your find-ings, you may require further investigations to confirm your diagnosis. You may wish to comment that you would like an arterial or venous Duplex scan

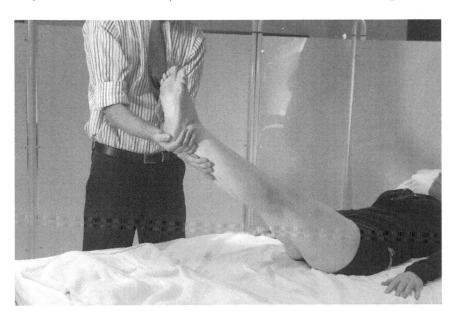

FIGURE A9.1 Buerger's test

or a computer tomography (CT) angiogram to confirm your findings.

If, during your examination, you find that a patient has arterial insufficiency, you should state that you would also like to do an ankle–brachial pressure index (ABPI).

To do an ABPI, ideally the patient should be laying supine at rest for 5 minutes. You will need a Doppler probe, a manual sphygmomanometer and some conductive jelly.

- Put the blood pressure cuff around the patient's arm.
- Using the Doppler probe, put a small amount of conductive jelly on the end of the probe and palpate for the brachial pulse. Once found, put the Doppler probe onto the area of maximum pulsation and listen for the Doppler waves.
- Pump up the blood pressure cuff until you can no longer hear the Doppler waveform.
- Slowly deflate the cuff, noting when you hear the Doppler waveform return.
- Repeat this on the other arm, taking the higher of the two brachial readings.
- Repeat the exercise, this time with the blood pressure cuff around the patient's leg. Find the pressure of both the posterior tibial and the dorsalis pedis, again, taking the higher of the two pressures.
- Check the pressures of the dorsalis pedis and posterior tibial in the other leg.
- Divide the higher ankle pressure of each leg by the higher of the two brachial pressures.

A normal ABPI should be 1.0. If there is arterial insufficiency, the ABPI will be less than 1.0, unless the patient is diabetic in which case you may not be able to compress the arteries (due to calcification) and this leads to falsely reassuring ABPIs.

Ensure that you have covered the patient appropriately and that they are comfortable. Thank the patient. Wash your hands.

Conclusion and presentation

Take a few moments to organise your thoughts before presenting your findings. You should comment on any pertinent positives or negatives from your findings. Offer a diagnosis.

An example of your presentation would be:

This is a 74-year-old gentleman who looks well and comfortable at rest. There is an insulin pen and glucometer at the bedside. On inspection, the left 4th and 5th toes have been amputated, with well-healed scars. On the left heel there is a well-demarcated, dry area of black necrotic tissue measuring approximately 4 cm by 3 cm. The surrounding skin is intact and pale. The left foot is cold to touch, with absent dorsalis pedis and posterior tibial pulses. The right dorsalis pedis is also absent. All other pulses are present. Buerger's test was positive on the left and negative on the right. In conclusion, this gentleman has a critically ischaemic left leg with non-viable tissue over the left heel. I would like to complete the examination by doing ABPIs on this patient.

Example of a vascular examination mark scheme

Before you start
- Makes introduction (full name and role)
- Offers explanation and seeks consent
- Ensures adequate exposure and patient's comfort
- Positions patient appropriately for each examination stage
- Washes hands

Examination
General, inspection and palpation
- Assesses general patient condition
- Enquires about pain
- Conducts a general inspection, noting any important points
- Recognises different clinical features of venous and arterial disease
- Makes a comparison of both sides
- Assesses capillary refill time

Venous examination

- Demonstrates knowledge of venous anatomy
- Examines patient standing and lying
- Conducts Trendelenburg test

Arterial examination

- Demonstrates knowledge of arterial anatomy
- Conducts Buerger's test
- Palpates all peripheral pulses
- Comments on importance of ankle–brachial pressure index in arterial disease

Completing your examination

- Covers the patient, ensuring that they are comfortable
- Thanks patient
- Washes hands
- Demonstrates empathy
- Presents examination findings in a concise and confident manner
- Offers (differential) diagnosis
- Does the above in a fluent, professional manner

10

Gait, arms, legs, spine

Introduction

Gait, arms, legs, spine (GALS) is a useful screening examination of the locomotor system. It is a general examination that enables you to identify areas of the musculoskeletal system that warrant further examination, and possibly investigation. For example, an individual may not have full range of movement of the shoulder, during your GALS screening. This will prompt you to conduct a full examination of the shoulder in an attempt to further explore the functional deficit.

Before you start

Read the instructions in full as they may be looking for you to conduct the GALS examination and find an abnormality that you need to examine further. Failure to examine the abnormality in detail could be severely detrimental to your final mark.

Enter that station and introduce yourself to both the patient and examiner. Gain verbal consent. Wash your hands and ensure that the patient is adequately exposed. Ideally, you will require the patient to be exposed down to their underwear.

Before the examination begins, there are three screening questions that you must ask:

- Do you suffer from any pain or stiffness in your muscles, joints or back?
- Are you able to dress yourself completely without difficulty?
- Are you able to walk up and down the stairs without any difficulty?

Examination

Although it does not follow the acronym, the easiest and most systematic order to conduct the GALS examination is:

- gait
- spine
- arms
- legs.

Gait

Ask the patient to walk away from you, turn, and walk back towards you. Assess the gait for:

- symmetry of stride length
- heel strike
- leg swing through
- toe off
- symmetrical arm swing
- turn – looking specifically at its stability and fluidity.

As the patient is walking, you can comment on what you are assessing to the examiner. If you have any concern that the patient could fall, you should ask the examiner or an assistant to walk alongside the patient. Do not accompany the patient yourself, as you will not be able to assess their gait properly whilst doing so.

Spine

Once the patient is standing in front of you again, you can begin your examination of the spine.

- From behind:
  - look for a symmetrical posture. Look at the line of the spine for obvious scoliosis, and paraspinal abnormalities. Look at the pelvic girdle, and ensure that the iliac crests are level
  - gently press over the midpoint of each supraspinatus to elicit tenderness
- From the side:
  - assess the curvature of the spine for kyphosis or lordosis
  - putting your index finger on one lumbar spinal process, and your middle finger on the spinal process below, ask the patient to bend at

the spine and touch their toes. Your fingers should move apart while remaining on the spinal processes (*see* Figure A10.1). If they do not, this indicates that the flexion movement is not coming from the lumbar spine

- From the front:
    — ask the patient to touch their left ear on their left shoulder, and then their right ear on their right shoulder. Observe for symmetry.

Sit the patient on the edge of the couch to assess rotation of the thoracic spine. Ask the patient to abduct their arms so that their elbows are level with their shoulders. Get the patient to rotate their trunk to the left, and then to

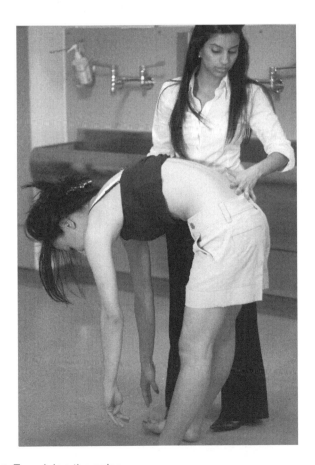

FIGURE A10.1 Examining the spine

the right. You can use their arms to assess how far they are able to rotate. Again, observe for symmetry.

Arms

While the patient remains sitting on the edge of the couch, ask them to extend their arms so you can inspect their hands. Observe elbow extension.

With the arms extended:

- inspect both surfaces of the hands, observing the anatomy and any deformities
- ask the patient to turn their hands over, to observe pronation and supination
- ask the patient to make a fist, to assess the power grip
- observe the patient's fine hand movements by instructing them to touch each fingertip with their thumb (opposition)
- squeeze gently across the metacarpophalangeal, proximal and distal interphalangeal joints, eliciting any bony tenderness
- watch the patient as you instruct them to put their hands behind their head and push their elbows back as far as they can, to assess arm abduction and external rotation (*see* Figure A10.2).

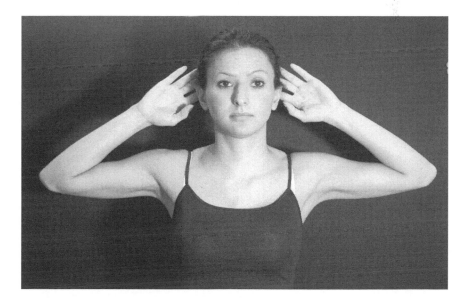

FIGURE A10.2 Examining the arms

Legs

Ask the patient to lie on the couch, then you should:

- one at a time, flex each hip while noting the range of movement and pain or tenderness elicited
- flex each knee, with one hand on the knee joint, to feel for crepitus; again, note the range of movement
- passively rotate each hip both internally and externally, noting limitation of movement or pain
- palpate each knee for warmth and swelling, before checking the knee for a joint effusion, with the patella tap test
- squeeze gently across the metatarsals, for tenderness
- inspect the soles of the feet, for callosities or ulcers.

Completing your examination

During the GALS examination, you may find some locomotor abnormalities. If this is the case, you may wish to further examine the area of abnormality by conducting a more focused joint examination.

Having completed the examination, cover the patient appropriately and ensure that they are comfortable. Thank the patient. Wash your hands before leaving the station.

Conclusion and presentation

Spend a few moments gathering your thoughts prior to making your presentation to the examiner, and offering a diagnosis.

Example of a gait, arms, legs, spine examination mark scheme

Before you start

- Makes introduction (full name and role)
- Offers explanation and seeks consent
- Ensures adequate exposure and patient's comfort
- Positions patient appropriately for each examination stage

- Washes hands
- Asks screening questions for musculoskeletal disease

Examination
Gait
- Observes patient walking and passes comment on their gait

The spine
- Inspects from three viewpoints
- Checks spine flexion and rotation

The arms
- Inspects hands
- Observes pronation and supination
- Checks power grip
- Observes opposition
- Examines small joints for tenderness
- Assesses abduction and external rotation

The legs
- Flexes hips and knee, assesses range of movement
- Rotates hip internally and externally
- Checks for knee effusion and crepitus
- Examines small joints for tenderness
- Checks feet for ulcers and callosities

Completing your examination
- Undertakes appropriate further joint exam
- Covers the patient, ensuring that they are comfortable
- Thanks patient
- Washes hands
- Demonstrates empathy
- Presents examination findings in a concise and confident manner
- Offers (differential) diagnosis
- Does the above in a fluent, professional manner

11

Shoulder and elbow

Introduction

Orthopaedic examinations are common in the final OSCE, because the patients are relatively well and examining them is simple. They represent a departure from the usual process of clinical examination (inspection, palpation, percussion and auscultation) and it is often more helpful to think in terms of: look, feel, move, X-ray. Be aware that the patient, whilst often systemically well, may have significant joint pain and it is important to be gentle and remain empathic at all times.

The station may start by asking you to perform the gait, arms, legs, spine (GALS) examination and then proceed to undertake a more focused single-joint examination. The GALS examination is covered elsewhere in this book (*see* Chapter A10, Gait, arms, legs, spine), so this chapter will focus mainly on the shoulder and, to a lesser extent, the elbow.

Before you start

Enter the station, read the instructions, and introduce yourself to the examiner and the patient. Explain to the patient what you wish to do, and why. Gain their verbal consent and wash your hands. They should be positioned appropriately for the examination and, in this case, the patient will often be standing with the upper half of their body exposed. Female patients should keep their bra on.

Examination

The shoulder

Look

From each observation point, look for scars, swelling, redness and deformity of the joint when compared to the other side.

- Standing in front of the patient, look for:
  — deformity of the clavicles
  — wasting of the deltoid muscles.
- Standing to the side of the patient, look for:
  — swelling of the lateral aspect of the shoulder joint.
- Standing behind the patient, look for:
  — wasting of the trapezius muscles
  — normal position, size and shape of the scapulae. Ask the patient to press their hands against a wall, and look for winging – this indicates damage to the long thoracic nerve supplying serratus anterior.

Feel

Check whether they are experiencing pain in the shoulder, then feel gently, but firmly, around the entire joint on both sides. Pay attention separately to the glenohumeral joint and the scapulo–thoracic interface. Push your fingers gently into the space between the acromium and the clavicle, and into the anterior glenohumeral joint space. Palpate the humeral shaft and head by pushing your fingers into the axilla. Observe the patient for pain and tenderness. Feel for joint swelling consistent with an effusion.

Move

Standing in front of the patient, ask them to perform a series of shoulder movements (active):

- Abduction
  — Keep their arm straight and swing it out to the side, until it points vertically towards the ceiling (note that some external rotation is necessary for full abduction).
  — Normal is 170°.

- Adduction
  - Move their straightened arm across the front of their body, keeping their hand directed towards the floor.
  - Normal is 45°.
- Flexion
  - Keep their arm straight and swing it forwards, until the hand points towards the ceiling.
  - Normal is 165°.
- Extension
  - Keep their arm straight and swing it backwards, until the hand points behind and slightly towards the floor.
  - Normal is 60°.
- External rotation at 90° abduction
  - Move their arm out horizontally to the side, so it is perpendicular to the body, and parallel to the floor. Bend the elbow to 90°, with the palm of the hand facing the floor. Then lift the hand towards the ceiling, keeping the elbow in the same horizontal position. You may need to demonstrate this.
  - Normal is 100°.
- Internal rotation at 90° abduction
  - Repeat the instructions for external rotation, but the hand should now be directed towards the floor, whilst attempting to keep the elbow in the same horizontal position.
  - Normal is 70°.

For each movement, compare the range and ease of movement relative to the other side, and also what is considered normal. Observe for any painful arcs, difficulty in initiating the movement, and any 'trick' movements. When observing abduction, it is also useful to stand behind the patient, so that you can comment on the amount of glenohumeral movement versus scapulo–thoracic movement.

Once this is complete, ask the patient to relax whilst you take their arm and passively move their shoulder through the same movements. Pay attention for restriction in the range of movement and also for any painful arc of movement. Feel over the joint for crepitus.

The elbow

The elbow, like the shoulder, has a number of articulations. However, there is probably not enough to examine at the elbow to justify a full OSCE station. You might be asked to examine it along with the shoulder, or following a GALS screening examination.

Look

Inspect the joint, extended and flexed. Look for joint swelling, erythema and local deformity. Comment on the presence/absence of scars. The normal carrying angle should be observed (5–15°), and any deviation from this commented on.

Feel

Check the patient has no pain in their elbow joints. Feel for the epicondyles and olecrannon. Comment on the presence of tenderness over these. Gently explore the radiohumeral articulation (lateral aspect of the elbow joint), beneath the biceps tendon, and the ulnar nerve (which runs behind the medial epicondyle).

Move

Again, allow the patient to demonstrate the movements in an active fashion before you perform the movements with them passively:

- extension (0°) – the elbow should be able to extend to form a straight line. Up to 15° in hyperextension is still normal. This occurs in women more frequently than men
- flexion (145°)
- pronation (75°)
- supination (80°).

Completing your examination

Orthopaedic examinations in which abnormalities are elicited should often be completed by performing a simple and relevant neurological and vascular examination. Examination of the regional dermatomes and myotomes, and palpation of the distal pulses, and documentation of capillary refill are the bare minimum required.

Finally, cover the patient appropriately and ensure that they are comfortable. Thank the patient. Wash your hands. Comment on the need to X-ray any of the joints, if appropriate.

Conclusion and presentation

Spend a short time internally summarising your findings. Present to the examiner and offer a diagnosis in the following fashion:

> This middle-aged gentleman presents with monoarticular disease consistent with a left-sided 'frozen shoulder'. Movement is globally reduced. Internal and external rotation are particularly reduced and both are associated with significant pain. The right shoulder has a full range of movement and is non-tender. There are no abnormal findings in the elbows.

Example of a shoulder and elbow examination mark scheme

Before you start
- Makes introduction (full name and role)
- Offers explanation and seeks consent
- Ensures adequate exposure and patient's comfort
- Positions patient appropriately for each examination stage
- Washes hands

Examination
The shoulder
- Makes inspection of the shoulder (from three positions)
- Enquires about joint pain
- Palpates the shoulder joint
- Observes active shoulder movements
- Passively moves the shoulder through its full range

The elbow
- Makes inspection of the elbow joint

- Enquires about joint pain
- Palpation of the elbow joint
- Observes active elbow movements
- Passively moves the elbow through its full range

Completing your examination

- Undertakes appropriate further joint and neurovascular exam
- Covers the patient, ensures they are comfortable
- Thanks patient
- Washes hands
- Demonstrates empathy
- Presents examination findings in a concise and confident manner
- Offers (differential) diagnosis
- Does the above in a fluent, professional manner

12

Hip and knee

Introduction

All joint examinations follow the same format. Put simply this is: look, feel, move, X-ray. It is important to remember that when an individual complains of pain in a specific joint, this could be referred pain, or arise secondary to another joint. It is not uncommon for patients to complain of pain in the knee, which either turns out to be referred pain from the hip, or secondary to an abnormal hip movement.

Before you start

Enter the station, read the instructions, and introduce yourself to both the patient and examiner. Gain verbal consent to examine the patient's hip/ knee joint by explaining what will be involved. Wash your hands and ensure that the patient is adequately exposed. To examine these joints properly, the patient needs to undress to their underwear, which will enable you to visualise their hips, knees, legs and lumbar spine. If the knee is being examined in isolation, a pair of shorts will suffice. Ensure that your patient is comfortable.

Examination

General

Standing at the foot of the bed, look at the patient and answer the following questions:
- Does the patient look well or unwell?

- Are they in obvious pain or distress?
- Are there any walking aids around the bedside, or other paraphernalia that may indicate an underlying pathology?

Gait

Begin both joint examinations by observing gait. If you have any concerns that the patient may fall, ask the examiner or an assistant to walk alongside. Watch the patient as they transfer from the bed or chair to a standing position, commenting on:

- ease of transfer
- assistance or aids that were required
- whether they looked to be in pain.

With the patient standing, ask them to walk about 10 metres, turn and walk back towards you. Observe for and comment on the following:

- symmetry of stride length
- heel strike
- leg swing through
- toe off
- symmetrical arm swing
- turn – looking specifically at the stability and fluidity of the turn.

The hip

Look

With the patient standing, you can begin your inspection.

- Standing in front of the patient, look for:
  — a normal stance
  — symmetry of their posture
  — level shoulders – do they look parallel to the hips, and do these look parallel to the ground?
  — evidence of pelvic tilt
  — obvious deformities of the hips, knees, ankle or foot
  — muscle wasting.
- Standing to the side of the patient, look for:
  — normal spinal curvature
  — fixed flexion deformity of the hip with a compensatory flexion deformity at the knee.

- Standing behind the patient, look for:
  — normal spinal alignment or evidence of scoliosis
  — gluteal wasting.

While you are conducting your detailed observations, you must comment on general features, such as:
- scars
- skin changes – particularly erythematous changes overlying joints
- deformities
- swelling
- limb shortening.

Remember, you should compare one side with the other throughout your examination.

Feel

You must ask the patient if they are in any pain prior to touching them. Remember, you need to examine both hips.

Start by comparing the temperatures of both hips and lower limbs, commenting as you do so. Temperature differences are important. A warm, erythematous joint may indicate a septic arthritis.

Palpate all around the hip joint line for any areas of tenderness. Tenderness in specific areas may relate to an underlying pathology:
- greater trochanter (trochanteric bursitis)
- lesser trochanter (common with sporting injuries to iliopsoas)
- ischial tuberosity (common with sporting injuries to hamstring muscles.)

Move

One should assess movement by starting with the 'normal' hip. When examining any joint, it is important to put it through its full range of movement. Because the hip is a ball-and-socket joint, this involves a variety of different movements.

Start with the patient lying supine on the couch. Ensure that the pelvic brim is perpendicular to the spine. Ask the patient to perform the following movements (active): flexion, abduction and adduction, internal and external rotation, extension. Then invite the patient to relax whilst you move their hips in the following ways (passive):

- Flexion
  - Place one hand under the patient's lumbar spine. This will enable you to detect any movement of the pelvis rather than movement from the hip (Thomas' test; discussed later).
  - Flex the hip to its maximum, noting the angle; normal is 120°.
- Abduction and adduction
  - Initially, stabilise the pelvic girdle by placing your forearm across the anterior superior iliac spines.
  - With the other hand, fully abduct the patient's extended leg to the point that you feel the pelvic girdle start to move. Again, note the angle: normal is 45°.
  - Test adduction in the same manner by crossing one extended leg over the other extended leg; normal is 25°.
- Internal and external rotation
  - With the leg fully extended, roll the leg both internally and externally. Note the range of movement by using the foot as an indicator.
  - Repeat the internal and external rotation of hip with the hip and knee flexed to 90°. Grasp the ankle with your right hand. Move the ankle medially to test external rotation (*see* Figure A12.1), and move

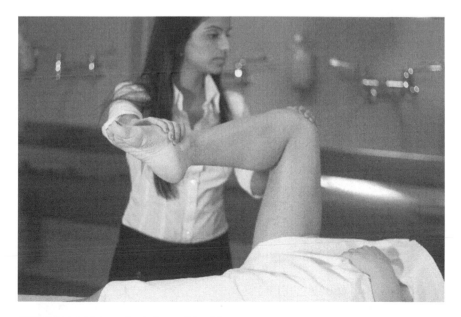

FIGURE A12.1 External rotation of the hip

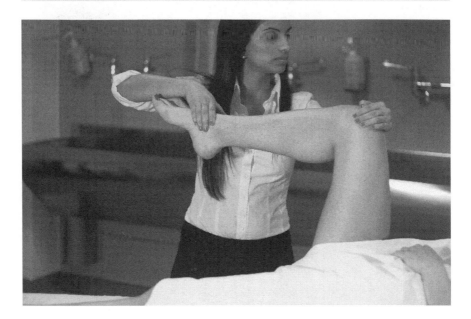

FIGURE A12.2 Internal rotation of the hip

it laterally to test internal rotation (see Figure A12.2); normal is 45°
for external rotation and 40° for internal rotation.
- Extension
  — Ask the patient to roll over so that they are face down on the couch.
  — Place your arm across the pelvis to detect any pelvic movement.
  — Lift the straight leg to assess the range of movement; normal is 20°.

Two tests that you may wish to perform are:
- Trendelenburg test – With the patient standing, ask them to raise one
  leg for 30 seconds, so that the knee is level with the hip. Repeat on the
  other side. The test is positive if the iliac crest on the side of the raised
  leg drops below horizontal. For example, if the patient's left leg was
  raised when the iliac crest on that side dropped, this would indicate
  weakness to the right hip abductors/gluteal weakness. It may also occur
  in osteoarthritis, due to pain.
- Thomas' test – If the patient has a prosthetic hip, this test should not be
  performed for fear of dislocation. Thomas' test measures fixed flexion
  deformities of the hip. Lay the patient on a hard surface. Place one
  hand, palm up, under the patient's lumbar spine. Passively flex both

of the patient's knees and hips as far as possible. Maintaining the non-test hip fully flexed (indicated by the loss of the lumbar curvature), straighten the other leg (test hip). If there is incomplete extension, this indicates a fixed flexion deformity. Repeat for the other side.

Measurement

It may become apparent during your observations that the patient has shortening of one of their limbs. This may be either:

- true shortening – where the actual length of the leg is shorter than the other side, or
- apparent shortening – where the actual limb length on both sides is the same, but the limb appears shorter, usually secondary to an adduction or flexion deformity of the hip.

You will need a tape measure to determine the nature of limb shortening. Measure the following distances:

- xiphisternum to medial malleolus on both sides – the apparent length
- anterior superior iliac spine to lateral malleolus on both sides – the true length

The knee

This is a complicated joint, frequently involved in rheumatological and orthopaedic disease. It may be examined in isolation or in conjunction with the hip. The patient can lie on the couch with their legs exposed (they should be wearing a pair of shorts).

Look

Observe, comparing both knees for:

- asymmetry
- joint swelling/effusion – limited to the area of the joint or extending beyond this
- bruising (trauma and associated ligament damage)
- scars and sinus tracts
- loss of supporting muscle bulk – suspected wasting can be confirmed with a tape measure
- varus/valgus deformity.

Feel

You must ask the patient if they are in any pain prior to touching them.

Feel around the entire joint space, commenting on any difference in temperature and noting any tenderness. Whilst flexing and extending the knee, identify the joint line. Feel medially and laterally along the length of the ligaments. Feel over the tibial tubercle for tenderness.

Perform a patellar tap test or fluid displacement test to confirm a suspected effusion. The patellar tap test is best for identifying moderate-sized effusions. Start superior to the patellar and gently but firmly slide your hand distally, emptying the suprapatellar bursa. Sharply tap over the patellar, and a 'click' will support the suspicion of an effusion.

The fluid displacement test is better for smaller effusions. Again, expel fluid from the suprapatellar bursa, and gently expel fluid from the medial side of the joint. Stroke the lateral side of the joint and observe the medial aspect for fluid filling.

Be sure to palpate over the knee whilst the knee joint moves, to identify any joint crepitus.

Move

The knee should be moved through extension and flexion, with both active and passive movement being assessed. As with the other joint examinations, pay attention to any restrictions in range of movement and any pain experience during movement.
- Extension
  - Instruct the patient to straighten their leg.
  - Normal is 0°, but hyperextension is fairly common, especially in females.
- Flexion (*see* Figure A12.3)
  - Instruct the patient to bend their knee (they will also need to flex their hip to allow this); normal is 135°.

One should now test the integrity of the supporting ligaments of the knee.
- Valgus instability – This will test the integrity of the medial collateral ligament. Place one hand on the lateral aspect of a fully extended knee. Push medially at the knee, whilst attempting to abduct the leg with your other hand holding the leg near the ankle. Compare both sides.

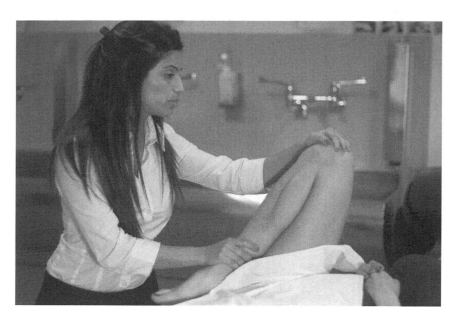

FIGURE A12.3 Flexion of the knee

- Varus instability – This will test the integrity of the lateral collateral ligament. Place one hand on the medial aspect of the fully extended knee. Push laterally at the knee, whilst attempting to adduct the leg with your other hand holding the leg near the ankle. Compare both sides.

Both of the above instability tests can also be performed with the knee slightly flexed. Significant joint space opening or instability may be associated with posterior ligament tears in conjunction with medial/lateral collateral ligament tears.

- Anterior drawer test (*see* Figure A12.4) (anterior instability) – The knee should be flexed to 90°, with the foot flat on the couch. Seat yourself next to, or just on, the foot. Grasp the upper part of the tibia with both hands, resting your thumbs on the tibial tubercle. Jerk the leg towards you and note any displacement at the joint. Compare both sides. Significant instability is consistent with an anterior cruciate ligament tear.

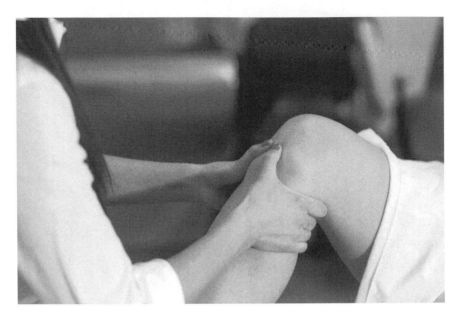

FIGURE A12.4 Anterior drawer test

- Lachman test (anterior instability) – Flex the patient's knee slightly, with support under the distal femur. Grasp the distal femur with your left hand and the proximal tibia with the right. Rest the fingers of your right hand over the joint and pull the tibia forwards. The test is positive if you feel the tibia shift forward with this action.
- Posterior instability – This will test the posterior cruciate ligament. Flex the patient's knee slightly, again with support beneath the patient's distal femur. Ask the patient to lift their ankle from the bed and observe for posterior subluxation. Then place your left hand over the joint and your right hand on the proximal tibia. Pull the tibia anteriorly and feel for it returning to its normal position. Subluxation and subsequent reduction indicates a posterior ligament tear. If the ligament is not torn, then simple downwards pressure on the proximal tibia may detect some degree of instability.
- MacIntosh test/pivot shift test (rotary instability/anterior subluxation of the lateral tibial condyle) – Extend the knee, internally rotate the leg and apply a valgus force to the knee. Next, flex the knee and feel for a jerk consistent with anterior cruciate damage.
- McMurray's test (meniscus injuries) – This test is performed with the

knee flexed and with the left hand over the knee joint to feel for clicks. To test the medial meniscus, rotate the foot externally and abduct the leg. Straighten the leg and feel for a click at the knee joint. To test the lateral meniscus, rotate the foot internally and adduct the leg. Again, straighten the leg, feeling for clicks. This examination is often not required in the OSCE situation, since it can be painful. It may be worth asking the examiner before you attempt it.

Completing your examination

Depending on your findings from the examination(s), you may wish to conduct a brief assessment of the lumbar spine. One can also comment on the possibility of undertaking relevant neurological and vascular examinations at this point. You may mention to the examiner that you would request plain film X-rays of specific joints, if you think they would be useful.

Make sure that the patient is adequately covered, and thank them. Ensure that they are comfortable. Wash your hands.

Conclusion and presentation

Present your findings to the examiner and include a diagnosis.

An example of your presentation may be:

> This is a 27-year-old gentleman who looks to be in significant pain and discomfort. He is holding his left leg in a fixed extended position and is in obvious pain. There are no mobility aids around the bedside. The skin overlying the left hip is erythematous and inflamed. The soft tissue appears to be swollen. There are no scars. The skin is warm to touch, with exquisite tenderness of the left hip on palpation. He complains of significant pain, and I feel it is unfair to ask him to stand. There is a severe restriction to both active and passive movement of the left hip in all directions. Inspection, palpation and movement are all normal in the right hip. Examination of the knees and lumbar spine is unremarkable. These findings are consistent with a diagnosis of left hip septic arthritis.

Example of a hip and knee examination mark scheme

Before you start

- Makes introduction (full name and role)
- Offers explanation and seeks consent
- Ensures adequate exposure and patient's comfort
- Positions patient appropriately for each examination stage
- Washes hands

Examination

General

- Makes general examination/inspection

Gait

- Observes patient walking and comments on their gait

The hip

- Inspects hips from different viewpoints and comments on abnormalities
- Enquires about pain
- Palpates joint, comparing both sides, and comments on findings
- Examines full range of hip movements, noting pain and limitation
- Examines for limb shortening

The knee

- Inspects knee, commenting on abnormalities
- Enquires about pain
- Palpates joint, comparing both sides, and comments on findings
- Examines for effusion
- Examines full range of knee movements, noting pain and limitation
- Tests for ligament instability

Completing your examination

- Undertakes appropriate further joint and neurovascular exam
- Covers the patient, ensuring that they are comfortable
- Thanks patient
- Washes hands
- Demonstrates empathy
- Presents examination findings in a concise and confident manner
- Offers (differential) diagnosis
- Does the above in a fluent, professional manner

13

Rectal

Introduction

Traditionally, the digital rectal examination (DRE) is performed as part of the abdominal examination. Reluctance on both the doctor's and the patient's part should not limit its clinical application and its importance should not be underestimated. It answers a great many questions, since many medical conditions manifest themselves at the anus/rectum. For example:

- a mass or fresh blood in rectal/distal colon cancer
- melaena in upper gastrointestinal (GI) bleed
- enlarged/abnormal prostate in benign prostatic hyperplasia/prostate cancer
- constipation
- fissures and fistulas in inflammatory bowel disease
- loss of anal tone in spinal cord compression.

It is very unlikely that you will have to perform the DRE on a real person in the OSCE, and mannequins are often employed. Remember to approach the mannequin in the same way you would a real patient.

Before you start

Enter the station, read the instructions, and introduce yourself to the examiner and the patient. Explain to the patient what you wish to do, and why. Gain their verbal consent and wash your hands. A chaperone should be present for this examination, unless the patient expressly declines.

The patient needs to be in the left lateral position, with their knees drawn up to their chest. Keep them covered with a sheet until you are ready to carry out the examination.

You will need:

- gloves
- gauze
- water-based lubricant.

Examination

- Put on gloves and gently part the buttocks. Inspect the anus for:
  — haemorrhoids
  — anal tags
  — fissures
  — fistulas
  — blood or mucus.
- Lubricate the index finger of your right hand. Ask the patient if they have any pain in the region. Place the pulp of the index finger at the anal verge. Check the lower sacral dermatomes by asking the patient if they can feel your touch. Warn the patient prior to insertion.
- As you insert your finger make an assessment of muscle tone. Also note any pain experienced by the patient.
- Fully insert the finger and note the presence or absence of stool in the rectum. If present, note whether it is hard or soft.
- Rotate the finger through 360°, making an assessment of the rectal mucosa. Feel for any masses/irregularities. Describe lumps as discussed elsewhere in this book (*see* Chapter A6, Lumps and bumps). In male patients, feel anteriorly for the prostate. Comment on its size, texture and the sulcus.
- Remove your finger and inspect for blood, melaena and mucus. Use a piece of gauze to clean excess lubrication jelly externally.

Completing the examination

Cover the patient and dispose of gauze and gloves in the bin. Check that the patient is comfortable and thank them. Wash your hands. Document the examination and findings in the patient's notes.

Conclusion and presentation

Summarise your findings to the examiner and offer a (differential) diagnosis.

An example might be:

> This elderly gentleman has normal anal tone and rectal mucosa. He has a smoothly enlarged, firm, non-tender mass anterior to the rectum. The mass has a central sulcus, consistent with that found on the prostate gland. There are no further findings related to the mass. The rectum contains no stool. There is no evidence of rectal bleeding or melaena. I believe this gentleman probably has benign prostatic hyperplasia, but we could further investigate this by measuring prostate specific antigen, and perhaps obtaining tissue for diagnosis.

Example of a digital rectal examination mark scheme

Before you start

- Makes introduction (full name and role)
- Offers explanation and seeks consent
- Offers chaperone
- Ensures adequate exposure and patient's comfort
- Positions patient appropriately
- Washes hands

Examination

- Makes inspection of the external area
- Enquires about pain, warns prior to insertion
- Inserts lubricated finger
- Comments on stool
- Examines the rectal mucosa through 360°
- Examines and passes comment on the prostate, if appropriate
- Removes and examines finger for blood and melaena

Completing your examination

- Covers the patient, ensuring that they are comfortable
- Disposes of gloves and gauze
- Thanks patient
- Washes hands
- Demonstrates empathy
- Presents examination findings in a concise and confident manner
- Offers (differential) diagnosis
- Does the above in a fluent, professional manner

Part B

Procedures

1

Venepuncture

Introduction

Venepuncture is a station where one can pick up some easy marks. It is also a station in which marks can easily be lost on silly mistakes. Many of us get into bad habits through laziness, and these are exactly the points that the examiner will be looking for.

Remember, if this station comes up in your examination, you will be demonstrating your phlebotomy skills on a plastic arm. It is advisable to practise this before the exam, since it is different to performing it on a real patient.

Before you start

Read the instructions, enter the station, and introduce yourself to the patient/plastic arm, and examiner. Explain the procedure to the patient and gain their verbal consent. Many people have gone for blood tests before, and it is therefore worth clarifying if the patient knows what to expect. If they have not previously had a blood test, be sure to explain that some mild pain will be experienced.

Ensure that you have the correct patient by asking them to confirm their name and date of birth. Check this with their wrist identity band, if they are wearing one. Prepare your equipment and wash your hands.

Equipment

You will need the following:

- needle of appropriate size
- syringe or Vacutainer® needle holder
- correct blood bottles
- alcohol skin wipe or chlorhexidine spray
- gauze
- sticking tape
- tourniquet
- gloves
- sharps bin.

Assemble the needle and syringe or Vacutainer® system prior to looking for a suitable vein. While doing this, you can ask the patient to roll up their sleeve to above the elbow, so as to expose the antecubital fossa.

Procedure

Ensure that the patient is comfortable before starting. Put your gloves on, and put the tourniquet around the patient's arm, approximately 10–15 cm above the antecubital fossa. Explain to the patient that this may feel a little tight, but should not hurt. Gently palpate the antecubital fossa for a suitable sized vein to puncture.

Use an alcohol wipe to clean the area. Explain to the examiner that you would ideally wait approximately 30 seconds for the alcohol to dry. Once you have cleaned the area, you must not touch it again, as this is supposed to be an aseptic procedure.

Ensure that all of your equipment is to hand, pick up your needle and syringe, and explain to the patient that you are about to take the blood. Then proceed to:

- anchor the vein with your free hand
- insert the needle at an angle of approximately 45°, with the bevel facing up. Just prior to the insertion of the needle, warn the patient by telling them to expect a 'sting'
- observe for a flashback, before drawing up blood
- ensure that your patient is comfortable and not about to faint
- having drawn blood, release the tourniquet
- holding a piece of gauze over the puncture site, withdraw the needle
- dispose of your sharp immediately

- ask the patient to press firmly on the gauze, to reduce bruising
- transfer the blood into the bottles, if not using a closed-system Vacutainer® device. Remember to take the tops off the bottles. *Do not* stab the needle through the top of the bottle
- fill in the patient details on all sample bottles
- put a fresh piece of gauze on the patient's arm, ensuring that the bleeding has stopped, and secure the gauze in place with a piece of tape.

To finish

Ensure that the patient is comfortable, and thank them. Clear up all of the equipment and dispose of it in an appropriate manner. Wash your hands. Advise the patient against carrying anything heavy with that arm for the next hour, to reduce the likelihood of bruising.

Example of a venepuncture mark scheme

Before you start

- Makes introduction (full name and role)
- Offers explanation and seeks consent
- Confirms patient's identity (name and date of birth)
- Ensures adequate exposure and patient's comfort
- Gathers appropriate equipment for venepuncture
- Washes hands and puts on gloves

Procedure

- Applies tourniquet
- Palpates for a suitable vein
- Swabs area and maintains sterility
- Warns patient prior to insertion of needle
- Obtains blood
- Releases tourniquet prior to withdrawal of needle
- Disposes of sharp in sharps bin
- Safely transfers blood into appropriate blood containers

- Fills in patient details on blood bottles (name, date of birth and hospital number)
- Clears away and disposes of equipment appropriately
- Thanks patient
- Washes hands
- Demonstrates empathy
- Does the above in a fluent, professional manner

2

Cannulation

Introduction

Cannulation or intravenous (IV) access is the 'bread and butter' of junior doctors' procedural skills. There are a number of indications for a patient to have IV access, and a non-exhaustive list includes:

- requirement for IV fluids or medication
- surgical or endoscopic procedures
- some radiological investigations requiring contrast media
- cardiac arrest or peri-arrest situations.

However, patients are often left with cannulas in-situ for days, which puts them at risk of local infection, thrombophlebitis and sepsis. It is therefore not only essential to have the skill to place a cannula, but also to have the sense to review them frequently.

In almost all OSCE stations that test ability to cannulate, you will be performing the skill on a plastic arm. It is essential, however, to do as you would if you were placing a cannula in a real patient.

Before you start

Read the instructions and enter the station. Introduce yourself and confirm the patient's identity, using their hospital wristband. Explain what you want to do and why it is necessary. Explain that it will be painful but that the discomfort will be short-lived. Gain verbal consent. Prepare your equipment and wash your hands.

Equipment

Prepare a small tray with:

- gloves
- cannula (appropriate size depending on indication)
- adhesive cannula dressing
- alcohol skin wipe or chlorhexidine spray
- gauze
- 5 mL syringe
- 5 mL normal saline (check expiry date)
- sharps bin.

Procedure (*see* Figure B2.1)

- Apply tourniquet, ideally to the non-dominant arm.
- Select a suitable vein through palpation and sight. Check its course to ensure that it is reasonably straight and not too tortuous.
- Put on gloves and sterilise the area with chlorhexidine/alcohol. Once this is done, it is important not to touch that area again. This is a sterile procedure.
- Allow chlorhexidine/alcohol to dry.
- Unsheathe the cannula.
- Hold the cannula between your thumb, index and middle fingers, making sure not to touch the shaft of the cannula. Approach the vein at 10–40° in the direction of blood flow (i.e. up the arm). Your thumb should be providing the force and, as such, should be positioned at the back of the cannula, over its rear port. Your index finger and middle finger should fall either side of the cannula shaft and hook lightly round the wings. This provides the 'steering'.
- Use your other hand to retract the skin over the vein, thus anchoring the vein in place.
- Pass the cannula through the skin and into vein. Arrival in position is marked by a 'flashback' of blood in the body of the cannula. Those with experience in placing cannulas will also feel a 'give' as you pass through the wall of the vein into the lumen. Ensure that you warn the patient just prior to insertion.
- Ease the plastic tubing of the cannula off the introducer and into the vein.

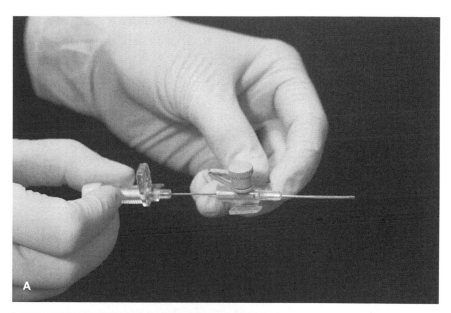

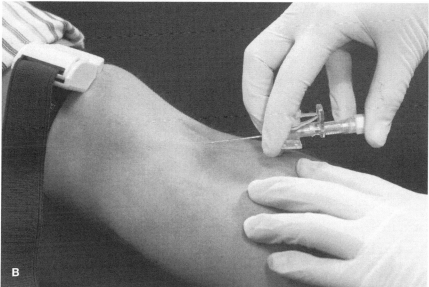

FIGURE B2.1 How to use and insert a peripheral venous cannula

- Release the tourniquet.
- Remove the introducer entirely, making sure to clamp the vein just proximal to the cannula tip and prevent blood leaking out. Place the introducer in a sharps bin.
- Apply the plastic screw cap to the rear port.
- Secure the cannula with a suitable adhesive. Write the date of insertion on the dressing.
- Draw up 5 mL of normal saline and flush the cannula through the top port. If it fails to flush or causes pain, it is likely to be in the wrong place. Remove and re-site elsewhere.

To finish
Clean up, placing items in the correct receptacles (sharps bins and clinical waste bins). Ensure that the patient is comfortable. Thank the patient and document the insertion. Wash your hands.

Example of a cannulation mark scheme

Before you start
- Makes introduction (full name and role)
- Offers explanation and seeks consent
- Confirms patient's identity (name and date of birth)
- Ensures adequate exposure and patient's comfort
- Gathers appropriate equipment for cannulation
- Washes hands and puts on gloves

Procedure
- Applies tourniquet to arm
- Palpates for suitable vein
- Cleanses skin and maintains sterility
- Holds cannula in correct fashion
- Warns patient prior to insertion
- Inserts cannula at appropriate angle, obtains flashback
- Releases tourniquet

- Threads cannula into vein
- Discards sharps (introducer) in appropriate container
- Replaces cannula cap
- Applies adhesive to cannula to secure it
- Flushes cannula
- Clears away and disposes of equipment appropriately
- Thanks patient and ensures their comfort
- Washes hands
- Demonstrates empathy
- Comments on need to document insertion and ensure regular review of cannula sites
- Does the above in a fluent, professional manner

3

Arterial blood gas sampling

Introduction

The ability to perform arterial blood gas (ABG) sampling is an important skill to develop before exiting medical school. It is an invasive procedure and is not without risks.

The arterial supply to the hand is provided by the radial and ulnar arteries. It is important to check the integrity of both components of this collateral system. This is done by carrying out Allen's test.

ABG sampling tends to be painful. As such, some people will use local anaesthetic for this procedure.

These points are important to recognise, however, practically, it is difficult to test this skill in medical school OSCEs. To do so would require a sophisticated mannequin or a very dedicated 'patient'.

Before you start

Read the instructions before entering the station. Upon entering, introduce yourself to the patient/mannequin and examiner. Explain the procedure to the patient and why it is necessary. Gain verbal consent. Remember to inform the patient that it will be painful, and give them the option of some local anaesthetic.

Ensure that you have the correct patient by asking their name and date of birth. If they are an inpatient, and the majority will be, you should check their hospital wristband. Wash your hands and prepare your equipment.

Equipment

In order to carry out ABG sampling, you will need the following:

- gloves
- sharps bin
- alcohol skin wipe/antiseptic spray
- gauze
- tape
- arterial blood gas syringe
- needle of appropriate size (23 G needle)
- local anaesthetic with needle and syringe, if required – remember to prescribe the local anaesthetic on a drug chart if you plan to administer it.

Allen's test (*see* Figure B3.1)

Although rare, one of the complications of radial arterial puncture is acute occlusion. If this occurs, and there is no collateral circulation from the ulnar artery, there is a danger of vascular compromise to the hand.

To conduct Allen's test:

- firmly press over the radial and ulnar arteries, with your thumbs on the patient's wrist
- ask the patient to make a tight fist and open their hand repeatedly a few times
- observe for pallor of the palmar surface of the hand, as blood drains from it
- instruct the patient to open their hand, and release the pressure of your thumb over the ulnar artery
- watch for colour returning to the palm of the hand
- repeat the test, this time releasing the pressure over the radial artery to ensure that colour returns to the hand
- arterial insufficiency is possible if colour fails to return to the hand, or is slow to do so – in this instance, arterial puncture should not be attempted on this side.

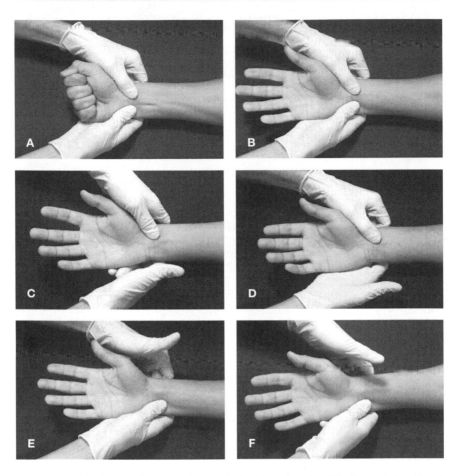

FIGURE B3.1 Allen's test. Both arteries occluded, fist clenched (A). Open fist, pallor of the palmar surface (B). Ulnar release (C), palmar surface of the hand flushes (D). Repeat occlusion of both arteries with clenched fist, then open fist. Radial release (E), palmar surface of the hand flushes (F).

Procedure

Assemble the needle and syringe (some kits may come pre-assembled). The syringe may be self-filling, or may require manual filling. It is important to be aware of both types.

Start by positioning the patient correctly, with their arm supported on a pillow, and their wrist extended to expose the anterior aspect of the wrist.

- Put your gloves on.
- Perform Allen's test.
- Palpate for the radial artery and identify the area of maximum pulsation.
- Swab the area of the wrist, allowing the alcohol to dry for approximately 30 seconds.
- Hold the needle and syringe like a pen. Approach at a 45° angle, bevel up. Insert the needle into the point at which maximal pulsation was felt (*see* Figure B3.2). Observe a flashback of blood. Remember to warn the patient prior to inserting the needle.
- Once you have collected approximately 2 mL of blood, hold a piece of gauze over the puncture site as you withdraw the needle. You must press firmly over the puncture site for 5 minutes. If the patient is able, they can do it themselves. If not, either you or an assistant will have to do this.
- Immediately after withdrawing the needle, stab it into the rubber block supplied with the blood gas syringe. Carefully remove the needle from the end of the syringe, and dispose of it in the sharps bin immediately.

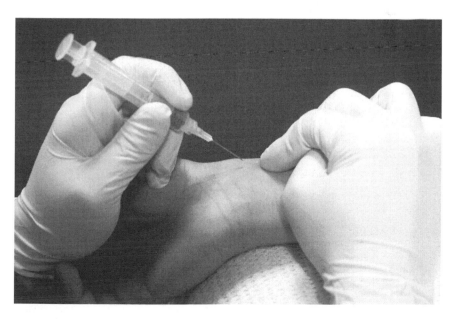

FIGURE B3.2 Technique for arterial blood sampling

- Ensure that any air is removed and put the air-tight cap onto the end of the syringe.
- Note the patient's temperature and the amount of oxygen that they are currently receiving. Label the sample with the patient's name, date of birth and hospital number.
- The sample must get to the blood gas analyser within 5–10 minutes. Therefore, someone should take it in person to the machine for analysis.
- Ensure that the bleeding has stopped, and tape a piece of gauze over the puncture site.

To finish

Ensure that the patient is comfortable, and thank them. Clear up all of the equipment and dispose of it in an appropriate manner. Wash your hands. Document the procedure, and put a copy of the results in the patient's medical record.

Depending on the length of time allocated for each station, you may also be asked to interpret a blood gas result. This station may be combined with discussion of, or use of, oxygen therapy.

Example of an arterial blood gas sampling mark scheme

Before you start
- Makes introduction (full name and role)
- Offers explanation and seeks consent
- Confirms patient's identity (name and date of birth)
- Ensures adequate exposure and patient's comfort
- Gathers appropriate equipment for arterial blood gas sampling
- Washes hands and puts on gloves

Procedure
- Performs Allen's test correctly
- Swabs area and maintains sterility
- Warns patient prior to needle insertion

- Obtains arterial blood
- Applies appropriate pressure to puncture site upon needle withdrawal
- Disposes of sharps appropriately
- Ensures that any air is removed from blood sample prior to attaching the air-tight cap
- Notes patient's body temperature and the amount of oxygen they are on
- Labels sample with patient's name, date of birth and hospital number
- Recognises time constraints and transport methods for arterial blood samples
- Clears away and disposes of equipment appropriately
- Documents procedure and records results
- Thanks patient
- Washes hands
- Demonstrates empathy
- Does the above in a fluent, professional manner

4

Male urethral catheterisation

Introduction

Male urethral catheterisation is a task often delegated to house officers and, as such, is commonly tested in OSCEs. In most hospitals, the nursing staff perform female catheterisation.

Catheters are often placed in patients unnecessarily and this exposes patients to infection and urethral injury. For this reason, it is important to establish clearly the indication for inserting a catheter and whether there are any alternatives. Painful urinary retention and shock are two of the emergency scenarios in which to place a urinary catheter. Less urgent indications may include chronic urinary retention, neurological injury/disease, and post-operatively.

Before you start

Read the instructions and enter the station. Approach the patient and introduce yourself. Check the patient's identity. Explain what you want to do and why it is necessary. Gain their verbal consent and offer a chaperone (it is often useful to have an assistant in any case).

Position the bed in a way that means you can be comfortable whilst performing the procedure. Position the patient so that they will be comfortable and on their back; legs slightly parted, knees slightly flexed. Preserve the patient's dignity by keeping them covered until you are ready to start the procedure.

Prepare a clean trolley, catheter pack (which may or may not contain gloves), a catheter of appropriate size, and a catheter bag. Open them all out in an aseptic manner, taking care not to touch the contents of the sterile packs. Wash your hands thoroughly.

There are two current variations on the aseptic approach to catheter insertion. The traditional method requires you to assign a 'dirty' hand, which holds the penis, and 'clean' hand, which handles the equipment. In recent times, there have been some OSCE scenarios that require a change of sterile gloves between cleaning the penis and inserting the catheter. Check which method your medical school expects. Aside from this difference, the actual technique of catheter insertion remains consistent. Whatever you elect to do regarding gloves, ensure that maintaining sterility is your primary objective and that the examiner knows this. We have approached catheter insertion in the traditional 'dirty' hand, 'clean' hand way.

Equipment
On your tray you should have:
- sterile gloves (one or two pairs)
- gauze
- plastic receptacle
- plastic forceps
- cleaning solution
- sterile drapes
- anaesthetic lubricating gel
- catheter of appropriate size (e.g. 14 French)
- catheter bag with connecting tube
- pre-filled syringe containing water for inflating catheter balloon (*do not* use saline, because it can crystallise in the balloon and prevent catheter removal).

Procedure (*see* Figure B4.1)
- Wash your hands thoroughly.
- Put on the sterile gloves.
- Ask the patient to lower their trousers and undergarments (ensure that they will be able to do this by themselves before starting, otherwise you have to do it as part of the preparation or have an assistant do it).

- Place the drape over the patient so that their penis is accessible through the central hole and is the only part of the body in the sterile field.
- You must now identify which of your hands is going to be 'clean', and which one is going to be 'dirty'. It makes sense for right-handed people who are positioned to the right of the patient to use their left hand as the dirty one.
- Pick up the penis in gauze (dirty hand). Hold it vertically. Retract the foreskin, if present.
- Using forceps and gauze soaked in cleaning solution, clean the penis, starting from the meatus and moving out and downwards. Dispose of each piece of gauze after a single use.
- Still holding the gauze-clad penis in the dirty hand, take the anaesthetic gel and inject a generous amount into the meatus. Allow a few minutes for the gel to pass down the urethra and exert its analgesic effects.
- After this short time period, introduce the catheter tip to the meatus. Feed it from the sterile plastic wrapping using a 'no-touch' technique. Insert slowly and feed along the urethra. Warn the patient prior to insertion.

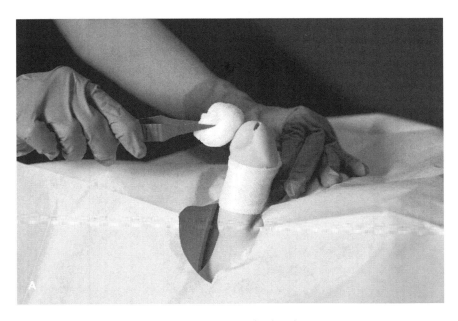

FIGURE B4.1 Preparation and insertion of urethral catheter

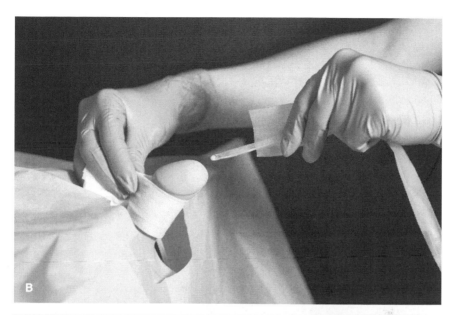

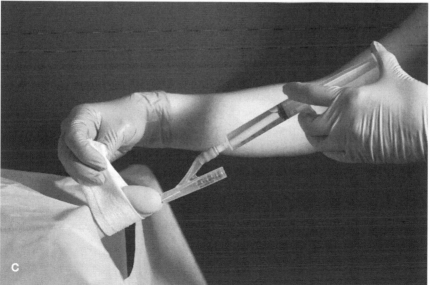

FIGURE B4.1 (cont.)

- You are likely to encounter the prostate gland at some point. Gentle caudal (towards the feet) traction of the penis should allow you to successfully navigate past the prostate.
- Continue to pass the catheter to the point of the 'Y' junction. Use the pre-filled syringe of water to fill the lumen leading to the catheter balloon.
- Once fully inflated, gently pull the catheter back until the balloon snags at the neck of the bladder. Ensure that there is a kidney-dish or suitable vessel for catching spilled urine.
- Attach the catheter bag to the main catheter lumen and hang in a dependent position. Clean around the patient and replace the foreskin, if present.

To finish

Ensure patient comfort and dispose of equipment appropriately. Restore their dignity, by covering them appropriately. Wash your hands thoroughly. It is essential to fully document details around catheter insertion. This includes:

- time and date
- consent gained, chaperone offered, name of chaperone
- catheter type and size (packaging often has stickers that can be useful)
- number of attempts and difficulty
- problems encountered
- residual volume of urine
- use or not of antibiotic cover.

Example of a male urethral catheterisation mark scheme

Before you start

- Makes introduction (full name and role)
- Offers explanation and seeks consent
- Confirms patient's identity (name and date of birth)
- Ensures adequate exposure and patient's comfort
- Offers chaperone

- Prepares appropriately, with catheter, anaesthetic gel, drape and cleaning equipment laid out on clean tray

Procedure

- Washes hands, puts on sterile gloves and drapes patient
- Holds penis in gauze
- Cleans around the glans starting at the meatus and working outwards
- Inserts anaesthetic gel
- Introduces catheter to meatus, warning patient prior to insertion
- Inserts catheter using sterile 'no-touch' technique up to the Y junction
- Uses gentle traction to negotiate the prostate
- Inflates balloon using pre-filled syringe
- Applies gentle traction to the catheter until the balloon catches at the neck of the bladder
- Attaches catheter bag and hangs in dependent fashion
- Replaces foreskin after insertion, if present
- Clears away and disposes of equipment appropriately
- Thanks patient and ensures their comfort
- Washes hands
- Demonstrates empathy
- Comments on need to document insertion, indication and residual volume
- Does the above in a fluent, professional manner

5

Ophthalmoscopy

Introduction

This is a difficult station because, like cannulation, it requires skill and dexterity. However, students often have had much less practice at ophthalmoscopy than they have at performing other 'tricky' procedures. Make sure that you are familiar with how to use an ophthalmoscope. It is always obvious to the examiner if you have not examined many patients' eyes. Examiners like to see someone who is confident with handling the ophthalmoscope, and want to hear you clicking through the lenses whilst you are examining the patient.

The eyes should first be examined undilated to visualise the pupils and iris, and then dilated to examine the lens, vitreous and retina. You should be aware that many patients and clinicians have refractive errors that will influence the lens selection used to visualise different parts of the ocular anatomy. For example, to examine a patient's retina, you will not always use the same lens; it will vary from patient to patient.

In this station, you may get either a mannequin or a real patient. There are plenty of patients around with hypertensive or diabetic retinopathy, so make sure that you are familiar with the different stages of both, as well as other common eye conditions. You may be shown images of a patient's retina, and be asked to comment on it.

Before you start

Read the instructions and enter the station. Introduce yourself to the examiner and patient. Gain verbal consent by explaining to the patient what the procedure involves. Some important points to cover in your explanation are:

- you will be shining a bright light in their eyes
- it may be uncomfortable but should not be painful
- they will be asked to focus their vision on a fixed point in the distance
- throughout the exam, they should blink and breathe as normal
- you will come in quite close and in front of their line of vision – they need to try to keep their eye focused in the distance
- check that the patient does not have a history of glaucoma if you are going to dilate their eyes (e.g. with tropicamide), and inform them that they should not drive or use machinery until the effect of dilation has completely worn off. This can take several hours. Remember, all drugs need to be prescribed.

Wash your hands and pick up the ophthalmoscope. Ensure that it works properly, and that the lens is set to zero.

Check that the patient is sitting comfortably, and inform them that you will dim the lights to aid the examination. Remember to tell the patient to let you know if they would like you to stop the examination at any point.

Procedure

The eye should be examined in stages, so that you do not miss anything. Examine one eye at a time from start to finish. If you are examining the patient's right eye, you should hold the ophthalmoscope in your right hand, and look though your right eye. Do the opposite for the left eye.

The red reflex, cornea, iris and lens

Start by looking at the pupils and compare them to one another. Ensure that they are the same size, and have a regular shape.

Ask your patient to fix their vision on a point in the distance. With the ophthalmoscope set to zero, look through it at the patient's eye, from about 1 metre away. You should observe for a red reflex, which is created by light reflecting off the retina. This is normal. Any abnormalities of the lens, such as cataracts, will appear black.

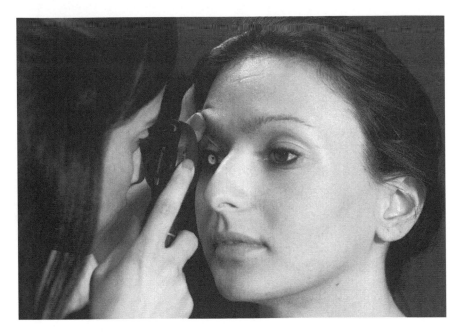

FIGURE B5.1 Ophthalmoscopy

From about 10 cm away from the patient, bring the red reflex into focus by moving through the lenses (*see* Figure B5.1). Again, you will observe abnormalities of the cornea, iris, lens or vitreous as black.

Keep clicking through the lenses until the retina comes into focus.

The retina

Once the retina has come into focus, you should clearly be able to see blood vessels. Follow these towards the patient's nose, until you are able to visualise the optic disc. You should then comment on the following features of the disc:

- colour
- margins
- cup-to-disc ratio
- blurring of the optic disc, if any.

Note the difference between arteries and veins. The arteries are relatively more narrow and pale than the wider, darker veins. Follow each of the blood vessels from their convergence point at the optic disc to each quadrant of the eye. During your inspection of the quadrants, you should comment on any abnormalities you find.

Finally, ask the patient to look straight into the light, to enable the visualisation of the fovea. This point is responsible for the highest visual acuity, and therefore any abnormalities such as dot or blot haemorrhages in this area warrant urgent ophthalmology referral.

Repeat the examination on the other eye.

To finish

Thank the patient and ensure that they are comfortable. Present any findings to the examiner in a concise manner. Wash your hands.

Example of an ophthalmoscopy mark scheme

Before you start
- Makes introduction (full name and role)
- Offers explanation and seeks consent
- Ensures patient's comfort
- If using tropicamide, ensures that patient does not suffer with glaucoma
- Washes hands

Procedure
- Positions patient appropriately
- Holds ophthalmoscope in correct hand for examination
- Demonstrates competent use of an ophthalmoscope
- Elicits the red reflex
- Adopts a closer position and passes comment on any abnormalities of the cornea, iris, lens or vitreous
- Identifies retinal blood vessels, following their course
- Examines all four quadrants of the eye
- Inspects the optic disc, passing appropriate comment
- Inspects the fovea
- Examines other eye

- Presents findings to examiner in a confident, concise manner
- Thanks patient
- Washes hands
- Demonstrates empathy
- Does the above in a fluent, professional manner

6

Otoscopy

Introduction

This is an unlikely OSCE station, but one that ought to be covered in limited detail. Otoscopy is the use of a light source and small speculum to examine the external ear and ear canal, up to the tympanic membrane. It is a simple procedure, but one that should be practised in order to demonstrate competence.

Before you start

Enter the station, read the instructions and introduce yourself to the examiner and the patient. Explain to the patient what you wish to do and why. Explain that it may be uncomfortable and that they should inform you if they want you to stop. Gain verbal consent and wash your hands. Check that you know how to switch the otoscope on before approaching the patient. The patient should be sat comfortably on the edge of the couch or in a chair.

Procedure

- Ask the patient if they have any problems with their ears or if they are at all painful.
- Conduct a brief examination of the external ear, noting the following:
  — discharge
  — erythema

— dry, scaly skin
— strong odours (particularly in conjunction with discharge).
- Proceed to examine with the otoscope. If you are examining the patient's right ear, hold the otoscope in your right hand.
- Hold the otoscope as you would a pen. In doing this, your ring and little finger will be free to press lightly over the patient's zygomatic arch (*see* Figure B6.1). This guides the otoscope in, and prevents it being inserted too far.
- With the left hand, apply light traction to the pinna of the ear, pulling it up and back. This straightens the ear canal and allows easier passage of the speculum.
- Look through the lens of the otoscope as it enters the ear canal. Warn the patient before insertion, and check their comfort upon entry. Note:
  — tenderness
  — redness
  — discharge.
- Observe the tympanic membrane. Comment on:
  — the triangle of light
  — perforation
  — swelling/bulging
  — effusion
  — discharge.
- Always ensure that you are looking through the otoscope whilst moving it inwards, as this prevents trauma occurring.
- Withdraw the otoscope gently, and dispose of the speculum tip.
- Repeat on the other side.

To finish

Ensure that the patient is comfortable following the examination. Wash your hands and present your findings to the examiner. It is very unlikely that the patient will have ear pathology, if indeed this station should arise in the final OSCE. It is more likely that you will examine a normal patient or mannequin, and then be asked to comment on a series of photographs of ear disease.

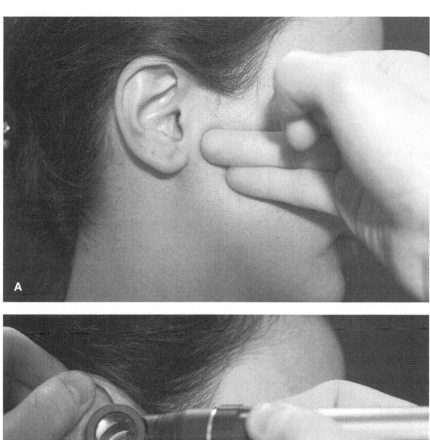

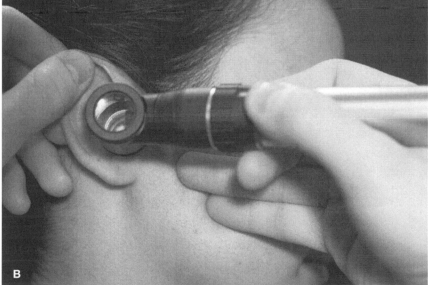

FIGURE B6.1 Technique for stabilising and using an otoscope

Example of an otoscopy mark scheme

Before you start

- Makes introduction (full name and role)
- Offers explanation and seeks consent
- Ensures adequate exposure and patient's comfort
- Positions patient appropriately
- Washes hands

Procedure

- Examines and comments on the external ear
- Demonstrates aptitude with the otoscope
- Warns patient before insertion into the ear canal
- Checks patient comfort
- Continues to look through the otoscope at all times whilst inserting it into the ear canal
- Visualises the tympanic membrane and comments on findings
- Withdraws the otoscope gently
- Repeats on the other side
- Clears away and disposes of equipment appropriately
- Thanks patient and ensures their comfort
- Washes hands
- Demonstrates empathy
- Presents findings in concise and confident manner
- Does the above in a fluent, professional manner

7

Blood pressure measurement

Introduction

The measurement of a patient's blood pressure (BP) is not, in itself, a difficult task. In daily practice, blood pressure is often measured using automated machines that have a high degree of accuracy. In the exam situation, you will be using a manual sphygmomanometer. Ensure that you are familiar with their use, including the use of different devices and the interchange of different cuff sizes.

Blood pressure, like all aspects of physiology, is very changeable and dynamic. Many factors determine a blood pressure at any one point in time. The anxieties of a visit to the doctor, a recent cigarette or coffee, or ongoing stress are just some examples of the factors that influence blood pressure. You must be mindful of these and other factors when recording blood pressure accurately.

Before you start

Read the instructions and enter the station. Introduce yourself to the patient and examiner. Check the patient's identity and gain verbal consent to take their blood pressure. Many people will have had their blood pressure taken before, and it is worth asking them before explaining the procedure to them. If they have never had their blood pressure taken before, you should inform them that although it may be uncomfortable, it should not be painful.

There are several questions that you might wish to ask before you take the patient's blood pressure:

- Do you take any blood pressure medicine?
- If so, what was the time that you last took your medicine?
- Do you smoke, and if so, how long ago was your last cigarette?
- Do you drink caffeine, and if so, when was your last caffeinated drink?
- Have you been at rest for the last few minutes?

Remember to wash your hands.

Procedure (*see* Figure B7.1)

Before taking a patient's blood pressure, you should leave them to sit at rest in another room for 5–10 minutes. Obviously this is not possible during your examination (or indeed often in clinical practice), but it is worth stating this to the examiner.

Select the appropriate blood pressure cuff for the patient's arm size. Incorrect sizing of the cuff can result in inaccurate blood pressure measurement. The cuff width should be at least 40% of the patient's arm circumference.

Once your patient has had sufficient time to rest:

- palpate for the brachial pulse
- once the brachial pulse is found, line up the arrow marked on the cuff with the arterial pulsation, and fasten the cuff
- ensure that the arm is supported, and is at the level of the heart
- palpate for the radial pulse on the same arm
- pump up the cuff whilst still palpating the radial pulse until you are no longer able to feel it. Note how many millimetres of mercury (mmHg) it takes to obliterate the radial pulse. Remember to warn the patient before you pump up the blood pressure cuff, explaining that the cuff will tighten around their arm
- let the cuff down rapidly
- feel once again for the brachial pulse, and place your stethoscope over the area of maximum pulsation
- inflate the cuff once again, to a pressure approximately 30 mmHg higher than the pressure required to obliterate the radial pulse
- deflate the cuff at a rate of 2–3 mmHg per second, noting the 1st

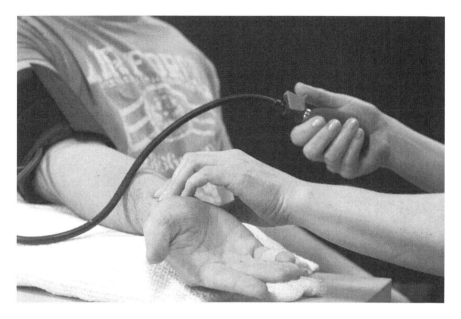

FIGURE B7.1 Blood pressure measurement

Karotkoff sound (the first audible sound). This marks the systolic blood pressure
- continue deflating the cuff at the same rate until the 5th Karotkoff sound (the complete loss of sounds), which marks the diastolic blood pressure
- let the cuff down fully and remove it.

To finish
Thank the patient and ensure that they are comfortable. Remember to wash your hands. Inform the patient of their blood pressure and record it in the notes.

When recording the blood pressure, be sure to include the following details:
- the systolic and diastolic readings
- which arm the BP was taken from (in some instances, bilateral measurements are necessary)
- the position of the arm, and the patient's position
- which cuff size was used
- if the patient appeared anxious or distressed

- antihypertensive medications that the patient is taking, and the time that they were last taken
- the timings of the patient's last caffeinated drink, or cigarette, if applicable.

When measuring postural blood pressures, you should start by measuring the lying blood pressure. Following this, stand the patient up, and repeat their blood pressure measurement. A significant postural drop occurs when the systolic pressure decreases by ≥ 20 mmHg and/or the diastolic pressure decreases by ≥ 10 mmHg, when the patient moves from lying to standing.

Example of a blood pressure measurement mark scheme

Before you start
- Makes introduction (full name and role)
- Offers explanation and seeks consent
- Confirms patient's identity (name and date of birth)
- Ensures adequate exposure and patient's comfort
- Asks appropriate questions – time of last antihypertensive, any caffeinated drinks etc.
- Washes hands

Procedure
- Expresses wish to allow patient to rest for 5–10 minutes
- Selects appropriate sized blood pressure cuff
- Ensures that patient is positioned with arm supported and at level of heart
- Feels for brachial pulse, and positions cuff correctly
- Inflates cuff while feeling for obliteration of radial pulse, then lets cuff down
- Whilst auscultating, re-inflates cuff to approximately 30 mmHg above that required to obliterate radial pulse
- Deflates cuff at 2–3 mmHg per second

- Identifies the systolic and diastolic blood pressure
- Documents blood pressure and informs patient
- Thanks patient
- Washes hands
- Demonstrates empathy
- Does the above in a fluent, professional manner

8

Nasogastric tube insertion

Introduction

Nasogastric tube (NGT) insertion is an important skill to possess, although in practice it is often performed by nursing staff. It is also not a comfortable experience for the patient, and as such, if you are asked to perform this procedure, it will most likely be on a mannequin.

Before you start

Having read the instructions, enter the station and introduce yourself to the patient and examiner. Check the patient's identity. Explain the procedure of NGT insertion and the reason. Gain verbal consent from the patient. Remember, an NGT is not always used for feeding. It may be employed for persistent vomiting and bowel obstruction, in which case gastric decompression will provide symptomatic relief. Some patients have had an NGT inserted before, so remember to ask them. This saves you from explaining something that they already know about.

Things to remember to mention to your patient are:
- the procedure should not be painful, but it will be uncomfortable
- it may make them cough or gag when the tube is being inserted
- if they want you to stop at any point, they should raise their arm.

There are some important contraindications to NGT insertion that you must be aware of:
- individuals who have suffered head trauma, maxillofacial injury or

anterior fossa injury warrant extreme caution – blind insertion of an NGT may result in passage though the cribiform plate, penetrating the brain

- individuals with a history of caustic oesophageal stricture or oesophageal varices also warrant extreme caution.

Equipment
You should ensure that the following is at hand:
- appropriate size NGT
- water-based lubricant
- cup of water with straw
- protective pad/towel
- gloves
- stethoscope
- 60 mL syringe
- sterile water
- kidney basin
- tape.

On occasion, it may be difficult to insert an NGT into a patient. There are a few techniques that may be employed in this situation.
- Put the NGT into the fridge for 20 minutes to make it less flexible, giving more control during difficult insertion.
- Ask the patient to sip water through a straw as you are inserting the NGT, encouraging the tube to go down the oesophagus rather than the trachea.

Procedure
Wash your hands before you begin and put on gloves. Start by ensuring that you have the correct length of NGT. This is calculated by measuring the distance from the nose to the earlobe, and adding it to the distance from the earlobe to xiphisternum. Mark this distance on the NGT with a small piece of tape.

Check the patency of both nostrils. Occluding one nostril at a time, ask the patient to blow out through their nose to find out which is the more patent.

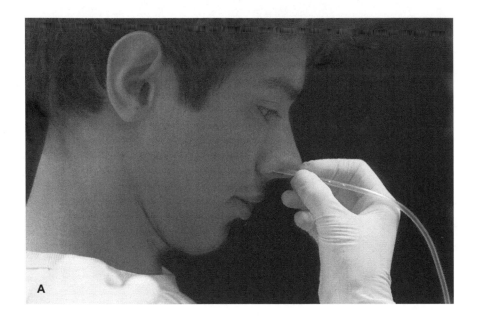

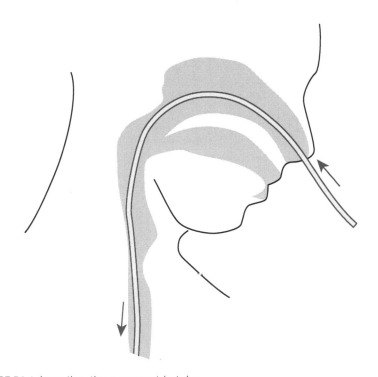

FIGURE B8.1 Inserting the nasogastric tube

Position your patient correctly, by asking them to sit upright and place their chin on their chest (*see* Figure B8.1). This position is the opposite of the positioning used to optimise a patient's airway in basic life support. The purpose of this is to encourage the NGT to enter the oesophagus, and not the trachea.

Put the protective pad/towel over the patient's chest, and hand them the cup of water with the straw. Explain to them that you will give instructions as to when they should start drinking the water. Have the bowl nearby.

With your patient comfortable, and correctly positioned:

- lubricate approximately the first 10 cm of the NGT with the water-based lubricant
- choosing the more patent of the two nostrils, start inserting the NGT into the nostril at 90° to the face, along the inferior nasal wall. Warn the patient before insertion
- once the NGT is in the pharynx, ask the patient to slowly sip water through the straw while keeping their chin on their chest
- continue inserting the tube until you reach the tape mark, at which point the patient can sit up more comfortably
- secure the NGT with tape.

To finish

Confirm that the NGT is in the correct place. This can be done by three ways:

1. using the syringe, aspirate some of the gastric contents; test the pH of the aspirate with litmus paper
2. inject a 30 mL air bolus quickly down the NGT whilst listening for a bubbling sound over the epigastrium with your stethoscope
3. obtain a chest X-ray – correct placement can only be confirmed if the tip of the NGT can clearly be seen below the level of the diaphragm.

Once it has been established that the NGT is in place, secure it with tape. Flush the NGT with sterile water, and clamp or connect the NGT as appropriate. Clear away the equipment and dispose of any waste in the correct manner. Document the NGT insertion in the patient's medical record. Ensure that the patient is comfortable and thank them. Wash your hands.

Example of a nasogastric tube insertion mark scheme

Before you start

- Makes introduction (full name and role)
- Offers explanation and seeks consent
- Confirms patient's identity (name and date of birth)
- Ensures adequate exposure and patient's comfort
- Gathers appropriate equipment
- Washes hands and puts on gloves

Procedure

- Correctly sizes up NGT
- Assesses patency of both nostrils
- Lubricates tip of NGT
- Correctly positions patient
- Warns patient prior to insertion
- Inserts NGT along inferior nasal wall
- Aids insertion by asking patient to swallow water
- Completes insertion and secures NGT in place
- Confirms correct placement of NGT, and is aware of various methods of doing so
- Clears away and disposes of equipment appropriately
- Documents procedure
- Thanks patient
- Washes hands
- Demonstrates empathy
- Does the above in a fluent, professional manner

9

Peak expiratory flow rate measurement

Introduction

Peak expiratory flow rate (PEFR) is a useful test that can be performed quickly and simply at the bedside. It is primarily used for objective monitoring of respiratory function in patients with asthma. PEFR is dependent on age, gender and height.

Many patients whom you encounter will already be familiar with the use of a peak flow meter, although they may not be using it properly. It is always worth asking the patient if they have ever used one before explaining the technique. Once you have observed them, you can then correct any imperfections in their technique.

Remember, once the patient has obtained one reading using the peak flow meter, they need to repeat the test a further two times. After the patient has produced three results, you select the best peak flow rate.

Before you start

The instructions for this station are likely to be relatively straightforward. Commonly, the station involves teaching a patient, who has been newly diagnosed with asthma, how to use their peak flow meter. It is possible that the station may also include either inhaler technique and/or interpretation of peak flow results compared to a predicted value.

Enter the station and introduce yourself to the examiner and patient.

Check the patient's identity and gain verbal consent from the patient in order to assess their PEFR. Wash your hands. The patient should be standing when they blow into the peak flow meter, and if available, they should wear a nose clip.

Equipment

In order to measure an individual's PEFR, you will need:

- peak flow meter
- new disposable mouthpiece
- peak-flow measurement chart, to record the result.

Procedure

Ask the patient if they have ever used a peak flow meter before. For those who haven't, provide a brief description of what is involved. Important points you should cover in your explanation are:

- the patient must be standing up
- the peak flow meter needs to be set to zero (*see* Figure B9.1A)
- the peak flow meter should be held so that the patient's fingers do not obstruct the movement of the slider

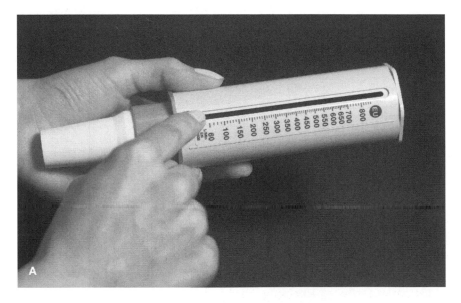

FIGURE B9.1 Technique for accurate PEFR measurement

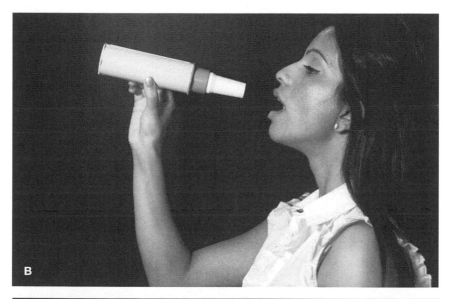

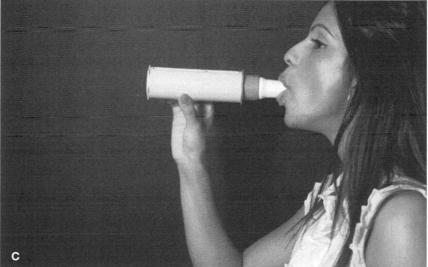

FIGURE B9.1 (cont.)

- next, a deep breath in is required (*see* Figure B9.1B)
- a tight seal should be made around the mouthpiece
- the patient should blow out as hard and as fast as they can – a good analogy is for patients to imagine that they are trying to blow out a

candle on the other side of the room (see Figure D9.1C). Explain that it is not a test of how long they can breathe out for, but a measure of how hard and fast they can blow out

- this should be repeated three times and the best of the three readings taken (the slider should be reset to zero on each occasion)
- the results need to be recorded on the peak flow chart and compared against the predicted peak flow based on the patient's gender, age and height.

Some patients will find it difficult to understand the description of what they are supposed to do. It is often worth demonstrating the technique to the patient, remembering that you must change the disposable mouthpiece.

Having explained the procedure to the patient, ensure that they carry out peak flow measurement. It should be repeated until it is done correctly. Invite any questions, and once answered, thank the patient.

Example of a peak expiratory flow rate mark scheme

Before you start
- Makes introduction (full name and role)
- Offers explanation and seeks consent
- Confirms patient's identity (name and date of birth)
- Gathers appropriate equipment for PEFR measurement (PEFR meter, disposable mouthpiece, chart)
- Washes hands

Procedure
- Explains that the patient needs to blow out as hard and fast as they can
- Ensures that patient is standing
- Ensures that patient's fingers are not obstructing the scale
- Gets the patient to repeat the PEFR three times, taking the best result of the three
- Demonstrates technique if necessary

- Repeat the procedure until patient is able to do it correctly (if initial three attempts were technically inadequate)
- Documents education and records results on peak flow chart
- Thanks patient
- Washes hands
- Demonstrates empathy
- Does the above in a fluent, professional manner

10

Inhaler technique

Introduction

This is another simple OSCE station where valuable marks can be picked up. It has a large amount of clinical applicability; asthmatics are in the hospital all the time and sound education regarding inhaler use can make a big difference to the severity and frequency of their presentations.

In order to add a layer of complexity, the patient will often be using both a short-acting beta agonist (blue inhaler) and a preventative steroid (brown inhaler). You must emphasise the roles of each.

- Blue (short-acting beta agonist) inhalers should be used on an 'as required' basis. They cause bronchodilatation through a mechanism of smooth muscle relaxation.
- Brown (steroid) inhalers should be used as regular preventative therapy. They are used in asthmatics that are requiring their blue inhaler regularly. A normal regimen for the brown inhaler is two puffs twice per day.

Before you start

Enter the station, read the instructions, and introduce yourself to the patient.

Explain that you have been instructed to discuss inhaler technique with them as a means of improving their asthma control. Invite them to demonstrate their inhaler technique to you. Take note of any deviations from correct technique, then explain and demonstrate how it ought to be done.

Procedure

The patient should be sat upright or standing. Explain that they should perform the following steps:
- shake the inhaler thoroughly
- remove the cap
- expire fully
- place lips around the mouthpiece, creating a tight seal
- begin inhaling through the mouth, and as they do press the canister down once
- continue to inhale maximally
- remove the inhaler, close their mouth and hold their breath for ten seconds
- breathe out gently
- repeat once more.

Invite them to show you what you have just taught. Once again, pay attention to their technique as compared to your own. Repeat the demonstration until the technique is well learned. If they still cannot perform the technique after a number of attempts, it may be appropriate to discuss a spacer device or alternative inhaler with them.

To finish

Once the technique is learned, it is important to reiterate the side-effects of using inhalers. One of the best aspects of an inhaled medicine is that it provides local drug delivery and limits systemic side-effects. Beta agonists can cause a tachycardia and tremor, which is worth mentioning to the patient. You should also advise patients to rinse/gargle with water after using the steroid inhaler, to reduce the risk of fungal throat infections and dysphonia.

Ask if the patient has any questions and answer these. Thank the patient for their time and reassure them that good inhaler technique is the cornerstone of tight asthma control. Document in the medical record that inhaler education has been provided.

Example of an inhaler technique mark scheme

Before you start
- Makes introduction (full name and role)
- Offers explanation and seeks consent
- Explains the importance of good inhaler technique
- Checks patient's understanding of the different inhalers
- Provides education as appropriate
- Checks inhaler technique

Procedure
- Comments on imperfections in technique (includes need to fully exhale, make tight seal with lips, begin breathing in, depress canister, inhale fully, hold breath for 10 seconds)
- Demonstrates correct technique
- Observes repeat attempts until technique correctly learned
- Offers further education on correct use of reliever (e.g. beta agonist) and preventer (e.g. steroid) inhalers
- Invites questions
- Thanks patient
- Demonstrates empathy
- Comments on need to document education provision
- Does the above in fluent, professional manner

11

Suturing

Introduction

There is a tendency for individuals who want to become physicians to ignore the skill of suturing in the belief that it is unnecessary, while the budding surgeons take time to hone their skills. Suturing is an important skill to learn, particularly when you start work as a junior doctor. Many wounds will require a few sutures under local anaesthetic in the Accident and Emergency department.

Ensure that you are familiar with some of the different types of sutures available. You should know the difference between:

- braded versus monofilament
- absorbable versus non-absorbable
- cutting versus reverse-cutting
- various size sutures.

If this station appears in your examinations, you will be demonstrating your skills on a mannequin. Many of these are not particularly realistic, and it is therefore advisable to ensure that you have at least some experience before the big day.

Before you start

Enter the station and read the instructions carefully. It is likely that you will be asked to demonstrate simple, interrupted sutures on a small wound. Introduce yourself to the patient/mannequin and examiner. Explain what the procedure involves and gain verbal consent. Important points to cover are:

- whether the patient has an up-to-date tetanus vaccination
- whether the patient has any previous adverse reactions to local anaesthetic or known drug allergies
- cleaning of the wound is likely to be painful
- injection of local anaesthetic may also sting.

Ensure that you have the correct patient by asking them to confirm their name and date of birth. Check this with their wrist identity band, if they are wearing one. Explain to the examiner that you would normally undertake a regional neurovascular examination before suturing a wound, to establish the extent of damage. Wash your hands, and prepare your equipment.

Equipment

In order to suture a wound, you will need the following:

- appropriate suture (type and size)
- suture pack containing sterile gloves, plastic receptacle, gauze, sterile drape, needle holder, forceps
- chlorhexidine/povidone iodine (for skin cleaning)
- local anaesthetic – check expiry date and ensure that you prescribe this
- 5 mL syringe
- needles (one to draw up the local anaesthetic, and one for infiltration of local anaesthetic)
- wound dressing of appropriate size
- sharps container
- a clean trolley for your equipment.

Lay out your equipment on the clean trolley. Open up the suture pack, taking care not to touch any of the contents so as to maintain a sterile field. Open the sutures, syringe and needles onto the sterile field. Pour some chlorhexidine/povidone iodine into the plastic receptacle.

It is useful to have an assistant present when suturing. You will need them to assist you with drawing up the local anaesthetic.

Procedure

Ensure that the patient is comfortable, and that the wound and surrounding area are adequately exposed. Before you touch the wound, you should inspect it and ascertain whether it is something that you have the skill to manage.

Explain to the patient that you will start by cleaning the wound area and will then proceed to inject some local anaesthetic before inspecting the wound more closely.

- Put on a pair of sterile gloves.
- Picking up gauze with the forceps, clean around the wound in a direction away from the wound.
- Create a hole in the sterile drape slightly larger than the wound, and place this over the wound to create a sterile field.
- Ask an assistant to hold the vial of local anaesthetic, upturned, while you draw it up into the needle and syringe. Check the expiry data and the contents of the vial prior to doing this.
- Change the needle for a new one.
- Infiltrate the local anaesthetic, warning the patient before doing so. Take care to anaesthetise the whole wound area.
- When infiltrating the local anaesthetic, you must pull back on the plunger to ensure that the needle is not in a blood vessel.
- Having waited a few minutes for the local anaesthetic to work, you should test the area to ensure that the patient is unable to feel anything before proceeding.
- Once anaesthetised, inspect the wound in more detail. Clean any debris from inside the wound. Observe for signs of tendon, blood vessel or muscle involvement. If these are observed, you should consult a surgeon.
- The wound can now be sutured.

When suturing, it is important to get good apposition of the wound edges and to ensure that the suturing is symmetrical. For this reason, you should start suturing from the centre of the wound. To place sutures:

- hold the suture needle in the needle holder
- gently part the wound edges with forceps
- insert the needle into the skin approximately 5 mm away from the wound edge

- release the needle from the needle holder, and collect the needle tip on the inside of the wound using the needle holder
- pull the suture through, leaving approximately 2 cm of the suture visible at the wound edge
- position the suture needle in the needle holder again
- insert the suture needle from the inside of the wound to exit approximately 5 mm from the wound edge on the other side
- release the needle from the needle holder, and pull the suture through to take in the slack
- holding the needle holder open, turn the long end of the suture around the needle holder three times, in a clockwise direction
- grasp the 2 cm end of the suture with the needle holder, pulling the knot tight enough to achieve wound edge apposition
- repeat the last two points, this time turning the suture in an anti-clockwise direction
- to complete the knot, repeat a final time, turning the suture three times in a clockwise direction to lock the knot
- repeat the interrupted sutures as many times as necessary
- lay all of the knots on the same side of the wound
- apply a dressing of appropriate size.

To finish

Clear away any equipment, disposing of any items in the correct receptacles, i.e. sharps in sharps containers. Ensure that the patient is comfortable, and thank them. Wash your hands.

Give the patient the following advice:
- as the local anaesthetic wears off, the wound is likely to become painful – prescribe some analgesia for when the anaesthetic wears off
- the number of days the sutures need to remain in, and where to get them removed – if using absorbable sutures, this is not necessary
- the number of days the dressing should be kept on, and how often it should be changed.

You should mention to the examiner that you would undertake a full examination of the vascular and nerve supply, including any tendons in the vicinity of the wound, prior to anaesthetising and suturing (*see* above). It is also important to document any neurovascular or tendon abnormalities in the notes.

Example of a suturing mark scheme

Before you start
- Makes introduction (full name and role)
- Offers explanation and seeks consent
- Confirms patient's identity (name and date of birth)
- Ensures adequate exposure and patient's comfort
- Comments on need to examine for neurovascular or tendon injuries before suturing
- Ensures no allergies to local anaesthetic
- Gathers appropriate equipment for suturing
- Washes hands

Procedure
- Puts on sterile gloves
- Cleans wound
- Maintains sterile field
- Draws up local anaesthetic, checking that it is in-date and prescribed
- Correctly infiltrates local anaesthetic into wound
- Explores wound and cleans thoroughly
- Uses correct suturing technique
- Completes suturing of the wound
- Applies an appropriate dressing
- Gives advice on wound care and analgesia
- Clears away and disposes of equipment appropriately
- Thanks patient and ensures their comfort
- Washes hands
- Demonstrates empathy
- Comments on need to document the procedure
- Does the above in a fluent, professional manner

12

Blood transfusion

Introduction

A station on blood transfusion may involve taking consent for and obtaining the blood, setting up the transfusion, or both. It is important to recognise that blood is a valuable resource and is in finite supply. As such, judicious case selection for transfusion is essential. Anaemia per se is not an indication, but patients who are symptomatic of anaemia (short of breath, fatigue, palpitations, tachycardia) are likely to be given a transfusion. Likewise, upper gastrointestinal (GI) bleeds and surgical patients may well require transfusion.

Blood transfusion is not free from complications, which is another reason for not offering this treatment without good indication. Complications range from febrile illness to septic shock, and haemolysis to chronic viral infection. It is important to be aware of these and monitor for them.

Before you start

Enter the station and read the instructions. Make sure that you understand what is required. Introduce yourself to the patient and examiner.

Explain the following to the patient:

- what you have been asked to do and why
- the indication
- the possible risks, and reassure them.

Wash your hands.

Equipment

You will need:

- venepuncture equipment (*see* Chapter B1, Venepuncture)
- cannulation equipment (*see* Chapter B2, Cannulation)
- Group and Save blood bottle and form (in most cases, there is a special blood transfusion request form that must be filled in by hand and signed by the person taking the blood and the person requesting the blood)
- gloves
- drug/infusion chart
- giving set
- drip stand
- blood product (once available from blood bank).

Procedure

Taking a Group and Save

- Whilst checking the patient's hospital wristband, ask the patient to state their name and date of birth (check these and the hospital number). This ensures that you are taking blood from the correct patient.
- Perform venepuncture (*see* Chapter B1, Venepuncture). Be sure to wear gloves throughout and safely dispose of sharps in the relevant container.
- Whilst still at the patient's bedside, fill in the blood bottle and blood transfusion request form, using the patient's wristband and their notes to ensure that the correct information is noted. If any of these sets of details fail to match, this will prevent the patient receiving the transfusion. Put your signature on both the blood bottle and blood transfusion request form.
- Prescribe the blood (number of units and rate) on the drug/infusion chart. In some cases, one might want to prescribe some furosemide to prevent fluid overload (normally 20–40 mg).
- Document the need for blood transfusion and the indication in the patient's medical record.

Setting up the transfusion

- The patient must have an intravenous (IV) cannula in-situ.

- Contact the hospital blood bank, once the blood is crossmatched, and request delivery to the ward.
- Prime a giving set.
- Once the blood is on the ward, the details on the bag should be checked against the request form, the drug chart and the patient's wristband. This must be done by two individuals.
- Record a baseline set of vital signs.
- Connect blood bag to the primed giving set, and start the transfusion.
- The transfusion of 1 unit of blood should not take greater than 4 hours.
- Observe the patient closely for the first 2 hours of the transfusion, with their vital signs being taken every 15 minutes.
- If you suspect that a transfusion reaction is taking place, stop the transfusion and disconnect the giving set. These need to be sent back to the laboratory for analysis. Any reaction should be carefully documented.

Ensure that you are aware of the different types of transfusion reaction, as the management varies. This will range from simply slowing the rate of transfusion to treating shocked patients with blood group incompatibility.

To finish
Clear away and dispose of equipment appropriately. Thank the patient and ensure their comfort. Wash your hands. Be prepared to answer questions on common transfusion reactions and how to manage these. Document details of the procedure the patient's medical record, if you have not already done so.

Example of a blood transfusion mark scheme

Before you start
- Makes introduction (full name and role)
- Offers explanation and seeks consent
- Confirms patient's identity (name and date of birth)
- Ensures adequate exposure and patient's comfort
- Washes hands and puts on gloves

Procedure

- Takes blood
- Labels the blood bottle and fills in request form at patient's bedside
- Prescribes blood on drug chart (considers need for furosemide)
- Ensures that blood is transported by appropriate means
- Ensures that cannula of adequate size is in-situ
- Demonstrates ability to communicate with laboratory when requesting blood
- Mentions two-person checking system
- Primes appropriate giving set
- Connects blood to patient
- Recognises time dependency of transfusion (4 hours)
- Mentions need to record baseline vital signs and then monitor vital signs regularly throughout the transfusion
- Clears away and disposes of equipment appropriately
- Thanks patient and ensures their comfort
- Washes hands
- Demonstrates empathy
- Comments on need to document appropriately
- Does the above in a fluent, professional manner.

13

Recording a 12-lead electrocardiogram

Introduction

This is a great OSCE station to get early on in the exam, because it is quick, simple and settles you down when your nerves are getting out of control. It is also an essential skill to be able to perform, since there are often occasions in hospital medicine where you may be the only person around to record an electrocardiogram (ECG).

Of course, once you've recorded the ECG, you need to interpret it, and this may well be tested in this station, too. Make sure you are aware of the following ECG patterns:

- normal sinus rhythm (regular with clear P waves followed by QRS complexes)
- atrial fibrillation (irregular with no discernible P waves)
- ventricular fibrillation (irregular and fast with disorganised electrical activity)
- ventricular tachycardia (regular broad complex tachycardia)
- abnormal lead placement/poor lead contact (appears as dotted line in relevant lead)
- ST elevation myocardial infarction and myocardial ischaemia (changes in ST segments and T waves)
- heart blocks.

The examiner may show you any ECG during the station and ask you to interpret it, but remember the majority of the points are for the procedure rather than the data interpretation. This station really is easy points if you just take your time and concentrate on lead placement.

Before you start

Enter the station, read your instructions and introduce yourself to the mannequin/patient. Check the patient's identity. Explain the procedure, the reasons for doing it and gain verbal consent. Wash your hands. Expose the patient adequately, whilst preserving their dignity. Ideally the skin surface should be clean and hair-free to ensure adequate electrode contact.

Equipment

You will be provided with:

- an ECG machine
- 10 leads (3 limb leads, 1 neutral lead, 6 chest leads)
- electrode stickers to go on the skin.

Make sure that the leads are connected to the machine, and that the machine is plugged in.

Procedure (*see* Figure B13.1)

- Attach the electrodes and apply the limb leads (these are coloured like traffic lights):
  — red – right upper limb (wrist or shoulder)
  — yellow – left upper limb (wrist or shoulder)
  — green – left lower limb (ankle, medial aspect of knee, or near to the anterior superior iliac spine)
  — black (neutral) – right lower limb (ankle, medial aspect of knee, or near to anterior superior iliac spine).
- Placement of these four leads will provide the traces of I, II, III, aVF, aVR and aVL on the ECG. Traces aVF, aVR and aVL are calculated as vectors of physical leads I, II and III.
- Apply the chest leads (these are numbered either C1–C6 or V1–V6)
  — V1 – right sternal edge, 4th intercostal space
  — V2 – left sternal edge, 4th intercostal space
  — V3 – 5th rib between V2 and V4

— V4 – mid-clavicular line, 5th intercostal space
— V5 – anterior axillary line, 5th intercostal space
— V6 – mid-axillary line, 5th intercostal space.

- Confirm lead contact and ensure that the machine is set to auto (as opposed to manual).
- Ask the patient to remain completely still for a few seconds.
- Press the record button on the ECG machine, and wait for the printed trace to appear. Briefly check its quality.
- Cover the patient adequately, without removing the electrodes, before reading the ECG.
- If adequate, remove the electrodes and allow the patient to get re-dressed.

To finish

Ensure patient comfort and thank them. Wash your hands. If you are likely to need serial ECGs, leave the electrodes attached to prevent lead position

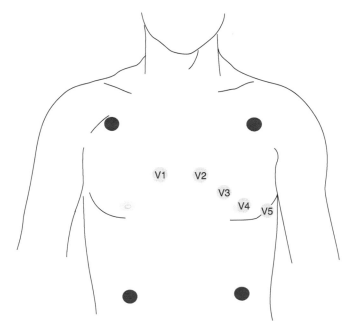

FIGURE B13.1 Positioning of ECG leads. Lead V6 (not visible) should be placed in the mid-axillary line

variations. Label the ECG with the time, date and patient details. Note on the trace whether the patient was experiencing symptoms such as chest pain or palpitations. Document your interpretation of the trace and sign.

In a 5-minute station, you will almost certainly be asked to interpret up to three ECGs at the end. Make sure that you are familiar with the common ECG patterns listed above.

Example of a 12-lead electrocardiogram mark scheme

Before you start
- Makes introduction (full name and role)
- Offers explanation and seeks consent
- Confirms patient's identity (name and date of birth)
- Ensures adequate exposure and patient's comfort
- Washes hands

Procedure
- Applies electrodes to correct places
- Connects leads carefully (makes effort to keep them uncrossed and not pulling on the electrodes)
- Asks patient to keep still
- Records ECG
- Checks quality of trace
- Disconnects leads (if appropriate)
- Thanks and covers patient
- Washes hands
- Records time, date and patient details on tracing, also documenting presence/absence of chest pain
- Correctly interprets tracing
- Demonstrates empathy
- Does the above in a fluent and professional manner

Index